CHRISTIAN BI

CHRISTIAN BIOETHICS:
A GUIDE FOR THE PERPLEXED

AGNETA SUTTON

t&t clark

Published by T&T Clark
A Continuum imprint

The Tower Building
11 York Road
London SE1 7NX

80 Maiden Lane
Suite 704
New York, NY 10038

www.continuumbooks.com

British Library Cataloguing-in-Publication Data
A catalogue record for this book is available from the British Library.

ISBN-10: HB: 0-567-03196-9
PB: 0-567-03197-7
ISBN-13: HB: 978-0-567-03196-9
PB: 978-0-567-03197-6

Library of Congress Cataloging-in-Publication Data
A catalog record for this book is available from the Library of Congress.

Typeset by Servis Filmsetting Ltd, Manchester
Printed and bound in Great Britain by
Athenaeum Press Ltd, Gateshead, Tyne and Wear

CONTENTS

CONTENTS

CONTENTS

PREFACE

A young discipline, the origins of bioethics are to be found in multi-disciplinary discussions about the practice of medicine in the wake of World War II and in the light of rapid medical developments in the second part of the last century. These were developments that not only caught the eye of members of the philosophical, theological and legal professions and of the medical profession itself, but they also attracted media attention and became subjects of public debate. Such developments included IVF technology and the launch of the Human Genome Project in the late 1990s. Bioethics became no longer an issue discussed mainly within the medical profession or by theologians and philosophers concerned with issues such as contraception and abortion; it expanded to cover many other issues than those discussed within the old confines of medical ethics. This meant that medical ethics in the traditional Hippocratic and Christian mould found itself challenged by a new more secular school of bioethicists, many of whom had been formed in disciplines that traditionally had had little to do with medicine. Today bioethics is concerned with issues such as animal research and ecology as well as issues more closely related to medical practice and medical research.

My own interest in bioethics goes back far. Both my parents were physicians. Although I did not study medicine, I was acquainted with the world of medicine from an early age. My youthful university studies were primarily in philosophy, first in Lund (Sweden) and then at postgraduate level in London. Later it was as a mother of four children that I came in the mid-1980s to work in the field of bioethics. Initially I worked as a researcher at the London-based Roman Catholic healthcare research institute, the Linacre Centre, headed by Luke Gormally. Subsequently I worked at the Centre for Bioethics and Public Policy, another London-based Christian institution. While at the former institute, I came in contact with the Guild of Catholic Doctors and had the pleasure of collaborating on a couple of books with Peter Doherty, the editor of the *Catholic Medical Quarterly*. At the Centre of Bioethics and Public Policy, now called the BioCentre, I worked with Nigel M. de S. Cameron, its Director and then the editor of *Ethics and Medicine* – one of the few international bioethics journals with a distinctly Christian profile. During these years I was also actively involved in the running of the European Association of Centres of Medical Ethics (EACME). As a member of the Association's executive committee I had an opportunity to work with many Continental bioethicists. Among them were notably Paul Schotsmans of the University of Leuven, who was for many years the President of the Association, and Guy Widdershoven of the University of Maastricht, the present President of the same Association, as well as the Italian bioethicist Emilio Mordini, who was also a member of the Association's executive committee in my days. Later I co-edited a book on nursing ethics with Bart Cusveller from the Lindeboom Institute, an EACME member and a medical ethics research centre in the Netherlands, and Dònal O'Mathúna, then at Mount Carmel College of Nursing, Columbus, Ohio. With my children nearly all grown up in the mid-1990s, I commenced doctoral research in the Department of Theology and Religious Studies at King's College London. This was under Michael Banner, then F. D. Maurice Professor of Moral and Social Theology and Religious Studies. While my doctoral thesis was on Pope John Paul II's theology of the body, bioethics has remained one of my central academic interests as a lecturer in moral theology at the University of Chichester and at Heythrop College, University of London – both academic homes where colleagues and students have provided a stimulating working environment.

Much water has run under the bridge since I started working in the field of bioethics some twenty years ago. The new reproductive technologies – and in particular IVF which made embryo research possible – were major issues when I started working in this area. Increasingly refined prenatal diagnostic methods was another important issue, and one in which I as a woman and mother took a special interest. Euthanasia was and remains a subject of much discussion, although today there is more debate about physician-assisted suicide, at least in the UK. Gene-therapy technology became a matter of concern in the early 1990s. There were fears about designer children made to order with qualities such as blond hair and special intellectual gifts. So far these fears have proved unfounded; most advances in gene therapy have been confined to cancer treatment. Insofar as we decide the characteristics of those who are born, this is done by means of prenatal selection. With the birth in 1996 of Dolly the Sheep, the first cloned mammal, cloning became a major subject of public debate. The hottest issue today is probably that of the creation of human-animal mixtures, that is, creatures that are part human and part animal. The status of these organisms, which are created by cloning for the purpose of being used for embryo research, is the subject of much debate.

While bioethics today embraces not only medical ethics but also issues such as animal welfare and ecology, the ethical and legal issues relating to medical practice and research remain central to the subject. Hence the larger part of this book is devoted to questions relating to healthcare and medical research. The last chapter deals, however, with ecological issues, while the penultimate chapter is devoted to questions about our relationship with animals. As regards medical regulations, I have given particular attention to the position in the UK, my home ground. This is especially in the area of embryo research where the UK has been in the forefront from a legal point of view.

A number of people have provided encouragement and helpful comments. Among colleagues, I wish to thank Helen Watt, David Jones, Peter Conley and Rosemary Cattell. Special thanks go to Katherine Treherne for reassuring me about the interest of the book. Catherine McIntosh and Sven Mauléon have also helped. I also want to thank Josephine Quintavalle and Teresa Iglesias. And I am much indebted to Michael Banner for his support at the beginning of my academic career. Most of all I thank Michael Sutton for his critical and patient encouragement throughout the year of this book's preparation.

This book is intended as an introduction to the subject from a Christian standpoint. It is aimed both at the informed general reader and at university students, typically perhaps those in their final undergraduate year or taking a taught postgraduate programme. It will have achieved its purpose if it promotes further interest in the increasing number of questions facing us in the field of bioethics.

CHAPTER 1

THE REMIT OF BIOETHICS AND TWO DIFFERENT APPROACHES

'These caves we call the lower regions. And we use them for coagulations, indurations, refrigerations and conservations of bodies. We use them likewise for the imitation of natural mines and the producing also of new artificial metals, by compositions and materials which we use and lay there for many years. We use them also sometimes (which may seem strange) for curing of some diseases and for prolongation of life . . .'

Francis Bacon, *The New Atlantis* (Bacon, 1989: 72)

INTRODUCTION: THE REMIT OF BIOETHICS

This passage from Francis Bacon's utopia, *The New Atlantis*, was written around 1624, nearly 400 years ago at the time of the dawn of science. Published posthumously a couple of years after his death, this work – Bacon's most prophetic writing – voices mankind's newly awakened scientific curiosity and aspirations. These are aspirations and a curiosity that have set their stamp on the modern world and brought forth new technologies affecting both ourselves and the world around us. Bacon's words express aspirations to prolong life and cure human diseases. There is a mixture of optimism and awe in this prophetic piece of writing – both equally justified.

Scientific development and technological progress have provided us with new comforts and many other advantages. Human society is being transformed by computer technology at the same time as advances in the biomedical sciences, not least in the areas of reproductive technology and genetic engineering, are making for new insights into the secrets of life, secrets which when revealed give us new possibilities to alter and modify various life forms from plants to animals to humans.

The frontiers of technology, science and medicine are constantly moving, making us ask more questions, giving us new answers and facing us with new problems. The new questions and problems are not only of a technological, scientific or medical nature, many of them are also of an ethical nature. That new knowledge and new-found technologies raise new ethical questions is especially true when they affect us directly as they do in the fields of healthcare and medical research. In these fields they affect our physical and mental wellbeing. Some of our new technologies affect our bodily integrity. Indeed, some of them raise questions about who we are and what we may or may not do to ourselves and future generations. In some cases they change our most intimate relationships, our sexual relationships and our parent-child relationships. Modern medical technology has made it possible to diagnose disabling conditions in the unborn child, thus facing us with difficult decisions in the face of the question of who should or should not be born. Medicine has always sought to alleviate suffering. But the question of whether we should prevent some unborn children from being born is new. That is, should we do so in order to spare them a life of suffering? The aim to avoid suffering remains the traditional one, but some of the means of achieving this end are beyond the remit of medicine in the traditional Christian and Hippocratic mould.

This is not only because new technologies present us with new options, but also because of a secular influence among bioethicists, physicians and others reflecting on the many issues now facing us within the field of medical practice and research. A new secular and utilitarian school of bioethicists is challenging the old Christian and Hippocratic school. Faced with technologies that allow us to make and unmake embryonic human life in the laboratory, this new more secular school tends to adopt a scientific and utilitarian as distinct from metaphysical and religious approach to issues such as the nature and status of early human life. The new technologies also allow us to prolong lives that would otherwise quickly perish. They make us question the value of human life when the quality of life is faltering. They confront us with the questions of when and how to die, just as they confront us with the questions of whether some unborn lives ought to be cut short because they might not be worth living. Our new technologies raise questions about the value of the human life both in its early and in its later stages.

Not surprisingly medical ethics has become a major issue in the forefront of public debate. Practices such as prenatal diagnosis, IVF and embryo research as well as end-of-life treatment concern not only medical doctors and patients, but society at large. They concern society at large, because these are the kinds of practices that make us question the very humanity of early human life, as well as the value of the lives of the infirm. Today, then, professionals from many different spheres of life are engaged in debates about questions of medical ethics. Politicians and members of the legal profession are called upon to make important decisions relating to questions of life and death. Scientists engaged in medical research enter the debates, often to defend their research. Theologians and philosophers and even non-professionals sit on advisory committees. Journalists write and talk about ever new discoveries and controversies. Even the public is consulted.

Of course, the questions raised by our technological advances, impacting on matters of life and death, reach beyond medicine and related areas of science. Bioethics therefore concerns not only medical practice and medical research. 'Bios' means life in the Greek language. Besides medical issues, bioethics concerns issues such as our relationship with other creatures and even our environment as a whole. They concern our world understood as our habitat, our source of sustenance, and a cause of joy and pleasure. Among the major questions of bioethics is the question of what we are doing to our environment. Are we going to leave behind us a world that is suffering the effects of pollution and wasteful use of natural resources? Not only is there the risk – to which C. S. Lewis pointed – that some men may sacrifice 'their own share in traditional human-ity in order to devote themselves to the task of deciding what "humanity" shall henceforth mean' (Lewis, 2001: 63), but there is also the risk that we will alter the very conditions for life in general. Some say that the greatest threat to us and other species might well be human-made climate change. Bioethics is concerned with the question of how we should care for creation in general.

TWO DIFFERENT APPROACHES

Bioethics is a young discipline. It started with a focus on medical ethics; and medical ethics remains its major concern even today. The roots of bioethics are found in debates that took place among scientists, doctors, lawyers, philosophers and theologians in the last century after World War II. The Nuremberg Declaration of 1947, which set out guidelines for medical research using human subjects, may be counted as one of the first fruits of bioethical reflection. The atrocities committed by the Nazis – though the Nazis were not alone in this respect – awakened a new concern about medical science. It raised questions about the remit of medical science and the role of medical doctors.

Later, as already noted, novel technologies in the second half of the twentieth century led to more questioning and a greater interest in what went on in medical practice. And secular influences provided fuel to the debates. Thus looking back, the American philosopher Tristram Engelhardt Jr wrote in his trendsetting work *The Foundations of Bioethics*, which was published in 1986, that 'the history of bioethics over the last two decades has been the story of the development of a secular ethic'.

One of the technologies that had a major impact was prenatal diagnosis with the help of amniocentesis. Developed to diagnose rhesus disease in the foetus in order to determine the need for early delivery, its main use was soon to be very different. It allowed diagnosis with a view to termination of pregnancy in case of foetal abnormality. This was a controversial issue at the time and it remains so today – as does the issue of abortion for any reason. Abortion on grounds of foetal abnormality, which has raised the question of whose lives are worth living, drove a wedge between the new more secular school of thought and the Hippocratic tradition of medicine dating back to 400 BC. It did so in a way that the debate about whether abortion was justified to save maternal life did not. For saving the mother's life could be seen as part of the healing aim of medicine in a way that termination on grounds of foetal disability could not. Thus the World Medical Association's *Declaration of Oslo: Statement on Therapeutic Abortion*, constituted a decisive break with the old tradition. It stated that, when there was a conflict between the pregnant woman and her unborn child, it was up to individual conscience to decide on an abortion or not, since 'there exists a diversity of attitudes towards the life of the unborn child' (WMA, 1970, paras. 2, 3).

Going hand in hand with these developments was a change of attitudes among patients. No longer content with a paternalistic approach among those who practise the art of medicine, patients

4

were increasingly voicing demands and asking for services. Demands for voluntary euthanasia were soon heard, although even today this is not an accepted medical practice anywhere other than in the Netherlands and Belgium. Physician-assisted suicide, on the other hand, which has long been legal in Switzerland and in the state of Oregon in the United States, is now being discussed in many countries, including England and Scotland. Today, then, patients often act as customers demanding services – and not only services that promote health or physical wholeness.

While both the old and the new medicine describe compassion as a prime medical virtue, and while both traditions are sensitive to human pain and suffering, they may advocate quite different approaches both at the beginning and end of life. The new medicine is prepared to shorten some lives in order to avoid pain and suffering. The old medicine will not contemplate killing a patient even for the sake of alleviating his suffering. If the Australian bioethicist Peter Singer, now at Princeton, is representative of the new medical ethics, the old tradition finds a staunch defender in the Roman Catholic Church. Singer is noteworthy by virtue of his international renown and the internal coherence of his position – once certain premises have been accepted. The Roman Catholic Church has been the most outspoken of the churches on questions of medical ethics and also the most coherent; and its most important spokesman has been Pope John Paul II, because of his concern with such questions and because of his twenty-seven-year pontificate, spanning a period when so many important issues rose to the fore. On John Paul II's understanding, 'life is always a good, a good of intrinsic value and sacrosanct' (John Paul II, 1995: para. 34). In Singer's opinion, on the other hand, 'the traditional view that all human life is sacrosanct is simply not able to cope with the array of issues that we face' (Singer 1995a: 189). Thus, while medicine in the Hippocratic and Christian tradition bans abortion, Singer argues that 'there are no grounds for opposing abortion before the foetus is conscious and only very tenuous grounds for opposing it at any stage of pregnancy' (Singer, 1995a: 209). To Singer's mind, 'life without consciousness is of no worth at all' (Singer, 1995a: 190). Hence, he has suggested that 'a period of twenty-eight days after birth might be allowed before an infant is accepted as having the same right to life as others' (Singer, 1995a: 217). And while the Roman Catholic Church and the Hippocratic tradition are firmly opposed to euthanasia, Singer would accept euthanasia at the patient's request. He would do so in the name of mercy. Thus in his book *Rethinking Life and Death*, from which I have just quoted, Singer sets out to overturn the old medical ethics. Arguing for 'a new ethical approach to life and death', he dismisses the principle of the sanctity of life espoused by the old medical ethics (Singer, 1995a: 189–90). Thus it is in regard to questions of life and death and the value of human life that the old school of thought and the new come face to face and clash. Hence a question such as that of whether the (human) embryo is a human being who deserves our protection is a question that drives as sharp a wedge between the old and the new schools of thought as do questions about abortion and euthanasia.

In the subsequent chapters, then, I shall often pitch Singer and his sympathizers against Christian voices, among them not least John Paul II. This will highlight the contrast between the positions taken by those engaging in the ethical debates from a secular and utilitarian perspective and those adopting positions in line with the older Christian and Hippocratic tradition of medical ethics.

While my sympathies lie with the medical ethics tradition of old, my aim is to give the reader a proper understanding of the different kinds of arguments that have been, and are being, presented for or against different medical practices and different types of medical research. So when in the next chapter I discuss the question of the status of the human embryo, I shall present arguments both for and against the view that the human embryo is a human being and as such should not be used in research.

HUMANS AND CREATION

Of course, the divide between the two aforementioned schools of thought relates to issues of medical ethics only. When we move to other areas of bioethics, we meet different kinds of argument and divisions. The question of the sanctity of human life is no longer an issue. But the question of suffering remains a focal concern. Indeed, it is the focal concern in discussions about how we should treat animals. With regard to questions about our relationship with animals it is also noteworthy that some of the protagonists in the debates remain the same as those engaged in discussions about medical ethics. Thus Singer, an advocate of animal rights, is again raising his voice against the Christian Church, and especially the

Roman Catholic Church. And yet as we shall see, in regard to attitudes towards animals, there is less of a difference between him and
the Christian tradition than he thinks. For the Judaeo-Christian
concept of stewardship sits well with a caring and compassionate attitude towards animals. It also sits well with concerns for the
environment and efforts to preserve a hospitable world for future
generations.

With respect to questions about the welfare of animals and about
ecological issues the divide is not between secular and non-secular
positions. Indeed, ecological concerns may be shared by people of
all religions and none. The biggest ecological question with which we
are faced today is that of how to curb global warming. If this is a
question that is engendering as much controversy as questions about
euthanasia do in medical ethics, it has also brought scientific thinking closer to religious thinking about human responsibility for the
world and about the interrelatedness of life. Unlike the major questions in medical ethics, many ecological questions unite people of
different outlooks to religion and to questions about the value of
human life.

That said, ecological questions about conservation of natural
resources and development of renewable sources of energy have
been linked to the question of population control to curb the accelerating growth of the world population. The last-mentioned issue is
one that is very divisive. Linked not only to different philosophical,
religious and cultural outlooks, but also to politics and economics,
it also reaches well beyond the remit of bioethics. Hence, as important as it is, it is not dealt with in this book.

Nor have I sought to speculate about the future and the questions
with which bioethics might be faced next. The present is giving us
enough pause for thought.

CHAPTER 2

THE BEGINNING OF LIFE

A squat grey building only thirty-four stories. Over the main entrance the words, CENTRAL LONDON HATCHERY AND CONDITIONING CENTRE . . . The enormous room on the ground floor faced towards the north . . . The light frozen dead, a ghost. Only from the yellow barrels of the microscopes did it borrow a certain rich and living substance, lying along polished tubes like butter, streak after luscious streak in long recession down the work tables.

'And this', said the Director opening the door, 'is the Fertilizing Room.'

Aldous Huxley, *Brave New World* (Huxley, 2004: 1)

INTRODUCTION: TO BE OR NOT TO BE A HUMAN BEING, THAT IS THE QUESTION

With the words above Aldous Huxley started the first chapter of his visionary work, *Brave New World*. They describe a building. Inconspicuous from the outside, it was housing laboratories in which human eggs were fertilized *in vitro* and gestated in machines providing the nutrients required for their growth. Some embryos were privileged and allowed to become single babies to be brought up as full citizens. Other embryos were divided to produce a cluster of clones. These cloned embryos were starved of oxygen to produce inferior humans, destined for the most menial tasks in society.

Huxley's work, published in 1932, warned mankind of the application of technology to the propagation of the human species. Fearing that this application of technology would be dehumanizing, he sketched a world in which humans were manufactured to specification and some humans allocated a higher intelligence and status than others. This was long before IVF was invented and long before anyone knew about prenatal testing or pre-implantation testing to avoid the births of sick and disabled children. Today Huxley's talk about ripened eggs and extra-corporeal conception and embryo selection does, however, not sound unfamiliar. We may not (yet) be substituting gestating machines for wombs, but we have already embarked on cloning. And while cloning for reproductive purposes is outlawed in the UK and banned by the United Nations, if the cloning technique is perfected, we may one day have human clones among us. Huxley's world would seem to be getting closer. And so we must ask ourselves whether we should take his warning seriously. Do the new reproductive technologies depersonalize reproduction? Are they an insult to human dignity? Do they respect nascent human life? Do they commodify the child? These are questions that will be discussed in this and the next three chapters.

It was the conception, successful gestation and birth, in 1978, of Louise Brown, the world's first test-tube baby, that first made various kinds of manipulation of the live human embryo possible. Her birth marked a new era in medicine, the era of extra-corporeal conception. The pioneers of the technology were Dr Patrick Steptoe, a gynaecologist at Oldham General Hospital, and Dr Robert Edwards, a biologist and physiologist at Cambridge University.

Theirs was a revolutionary achievement. But it set reproductive science at odds with many religious groups. This was not only because of the artificiality of IVF conception, though this made many people feel uneasy. To the mind of many philosophers and theologians, the most important consideration was the loss of embryonic life linked to IVF. In particular, it was the deliberate destruction of the human embryo in research that became the object of a heated debate. This then was a debate between those who saw such research as legitimate and those who considered embryo research on a par with homicide.

Of course, the media hailed the birth of Louise Brown as a glorious medical feat. But it soon unsettled many among the public, religious and non-religious. Yet today, few people raise an eyebrow when told about an IVF child; IVF is now a commonplace procedure. Nevertheless, each time we hear about new kinds of embryo research or of a new way of making babies in the test tube a debate flares up. These technologies and procedures catch our attention again and again. Why? Because they make us question who we are. They raise questions about our humanity and about human rights. They challenge us. They make us question what it means to be human. Some of us hail the new technological developments and procedures as human progress. Others warn that they are dehumanizing.

The IVF technology has created a fault-line between two camps with very different outlooks. One consists of those keen to improve extra-corporeal conception technology not only to overcome infertility but also to promote science and healing, using the embryo made available by being created outside the body. In this camp are scientists and their supporters who hail cloning for research purposes, so-called 'therapeutic cloning', with a view to finding new cures of human diseases, as a promising achievement. This camp is keen to meet adult desires and promote adult health interests. It insists on the need for embryo research in order to achieve the aforementioned goals. It does not regard the human embryo as a human being to be respected and protected. The other camp consists of all those bioethicists, religious bodies and others who worry about the wellbeing of the child-to-be and object to human embryo research, not least in the form of therapeutic cloning, on the ground that it involves the deliberate destruction of human life. The fear expressed on this side of the fault-line is that these new technologies foster an increasingly instrumental attitude towards the human embryo and child-to-be.

The main focus in this chapter is on the moral status of the early pre-14-day human embryo, and the justifiability of embryo research and IVF involving embryo wastage. This is an important issue, because today we can deliberately make, remake and unmake the human embryo in the laboratory. And it is legal to do so until the end of the 14th day after fertilization, when the primitive streak appears. The pre-14-day human embryo can be used in research in the pursuit of new cures for human ailments.

As to the justifiability of creating embryos of partly human and partly animal origin and the question of the status of these creatures, these issues are deferred until Chapter 7. Hence, the term embryo is reserved for the human embryo in the remainder of this chapter.

TO BE OR NOT TO BE AN INDIVIDUAL HUMAN BEING, THAT IS THE QUESTION

'It was you who created my inmost self and put me together in my mother's womb' (Psalm 139). The Psalmist wrote this long before *in vitro* fertilization was thought of and long before the advent of cloning. However, the line just quoted raises an important question. It raises the most important question of all in the contexts of embryo research and human embryo wastage. This is the question of when human, or personal, life begins. Is the human embryo created in the laboratory a disposable biological product? Or is it an entity that deserves our respect and protection?

On one line of reasoning, that embraced by many who consider the morning-after pill to be a contraceptive – rather than a means of abortion – the human embryo cannot be described as a human being before it has embedded itself in the maternal womb. Others say that there is no individual human life until the so-called primitive streak has appeared some 14 days after fertilization. The primitive streak is the first beginning, or precursor, of the neural cord and gives a longitudinal indication of the orientation of the embryo. Also, the embryo can no longer split in two and twin after the appearance of the primitive streak.

If, indeed, it is correct that the human embryo cannot be regarded as a human individual or a person until it has reached a certain stage, then objections to IVF on grounds of early embryo wastage lose their weight. So too do objections to research using the early human embryo. Thus if human life only begins at or after implantation, or at the time of the appearance of the so-called primitive streak or later, then the embryo wastage linked to creation of embryos *in vitro* is of little moral importance. If the early human embryo is but a blob of tissue, then research involving its destruction is morally unproblematic. In other words, if there is a crucial cut-off point in the embryological development at which human life begins, then until that point is reached the respect or protection we owe the embryo is limited.

If by contrast, the embryo created *in vitro* is from the very beginning a human being or a person and, therefore, deserves our respect and protection, then human embryo research and embryo wastage in connection with IVF are hard to justify. In order morally to justify human embryo research and the embryo wastage linked to IVF, we must be able to provide convincing arguments for saying that the early human embryo is not an entity deserving our respect and protection. Such an argument would be provided if we could show that the early human embryo is a mere aggregate of cells lacking proper human status and lacking even the status of an individual organism.

Here we shall look at a number of biological arguments for saying that the human embryo does not have a proper human or an individual status until it has reached a certain stage on its life journey. One of these is the argument that the embryo is not to be counted as a human being until it has implanted itself in the lining of the uterus. We shall also look at arguments in favour of pinpointing a certain stage of embryonic development and identifying it as that from which the embryo should be regarded as a human being or a person. In this context we shall briefly look back at the Thomist understanding of when the human embryo is sufficiently formed to house the rational and personal soul. We shall then consider the merits of the science-based arguments that were of seminal importance for the legalization of embryo research under the UK's Human Fertilization and Embryology Act 1990 (HFE ACT 1990). According to the last-mentioned type of argument, the early pre-14 day embryo – or fertilized egg – is not an individual organism, and so not an individual human being.[1]

IMPLANTATION

If human life begins when the embryo has embedded itself in the lining of the maternal womb, then neither the embryo conceived in the womb, nor the embryo created outside the womb, can be counted as a human being until this process, the process of implantation, has taken place. But how could a process such as implantation be a criterion on the basis of which to decide whether the embryo is a human being? The change that has taken place once the embryo has travelled down the fallopian tube and implanted itself in the womb is one of environment and nourishment. The claim that implantation radically changes the nature of the developing entity is not convincing.

Of course, implantation is a crucial stage in the development of the embryo. The embryo has to embed itself in the lining of the womb in order to receive nourishment. Unless implantation takes place it will perish. But likewise, the nine-month-old foetus must leave the restricted space of the womb to breath and receive new types of nourishment in order to continue on its life journey. Every living organism needs proper nourishment and a suitable environment in order to thrive.

That said, implantation marks the beginning of a new relationship. The novelty of this relationship is less obvious if the embryo is conceived *in vivo* (in the maternal body) than if it is conceived *in vitro* (outside the maternal body). But, in either case, as from the time of implantation the maternal nourishing begins. Meaning no offence, we might even say that at the time of implantation the embryo begins a parasitical existence: the embryo becomes uniquely dependent on its gestational mother.

Before implantation has taken place there is, at least in principle, a choice of venue for its continued existence. It is not yet uniquely dependent on a particular gestational mother. Of course, a thriving embryo conceived *in vivo* will normally implant itself in the maternal womb, that is, the womb belonging to its genetic mother. It could, however, be flushed out of the maternal body and given to another woman to gestate. In principle, it could end up in different venues. This is even truer of the embryo conceived *in vitro*. While it may be returned to its genetic mother, it could also be donated to another woman. Alternatively, it could be placed in storage for future fertility treatment, or it could end up in the laboratory as research material.

So implantation is an important stage in the embryo's life journey. But it has nothing to do with the question of whether the embryo is a human being or not. Implantation is the start of a physical bond between the embryo and the gestating mother and, usually, also the beginning of a psychological bonding process. The mother normally starts bonding with the expected child; so too may the father.[2] And so the expected child becomes increasingly recognized as part of the family. Implantation is the beginning of a special relationship with the gestational mother and her family.

ARGUMENTS WITH REFERENCE TO FORMATION

A quite different type of argument for not counting the early embryo/foetus as a human being or person is that based on its bodily formation and ability to house the human or personal soul.[3] This kind of argument is ancient. It is found already in the writings of the Greek philosopher Aristotle (384 BC–322 BC), and it comes in various versions. The one advanced by Aristotle was taken up again in the Middle Ages by St Thomas Aquinas (*c*.1224–1274 AD). Like Aristotle, Aquinas spoke of three types of soul: the vegetative soul, the sentient (or animal) soul, and the rational soul (Aquinas, ST, I, qq 74–78; ScG, Book ii, q 56). These souls, he said, possess different types of power. Thus the vegetative soul possesses the powers of reproduction, growth, assimilation of nourishment and excretion. The sentient soul possesses all the powers of the vegetative soul as well as the powers of locomotion, sensation and desire. And the rational soul possesses all the powers of the two lower souls plus the power of reasoning, hand in hand with which goes the power of the free will.

Seeing the soul of an organism as its life-principle, Aquinas argued that the soul of the human embryo/foetus goes through different stages, acquiring more and more capacities and potentialities. The first stage is the vegetative stage, the second the sentient stage and the third and last stage that at which the soul acquires the potential for rationality. According to this understanding, the soul is what makes the organism live and gives it different powers and potentialities. So even if it does not reproduce itself, the early embryo is alive with a vegetative soul, since the cells in its little body are multiplying and take in nourishment and excrete by-products. Later, with the formation of the required organs or structures of the body, the embryo foetus becomes alive with a sentient soul. But only when the foetal body is fully formed can the foetus be alive with a rational soul, a soul inherent in which is the potential to acquire the intellectual ability of rationality. Following Aristotle, Aquinas said that the male foetus is formed and ready to house the rational soul on the 40th day after conception, whereas the female foetus develops more slowly and is not ready to house the rational soul until the 90th day after conception. In other words, Aquinas linked animation, that is, the infusion of the rational soul, to the formation of the embryo/foetus. On his understanding, there was not a human person until the embryo/foetus was alive with a rational soul.

This line of thinking was no novelty in the Christian tradition, though it should be noted that there were two main types of animation theory among early Christian thinkers: the traducianist theory and the creationist theory. On the traducianist theory, animation was immediate and transmitted with the male seed. On the creationist theory, the soul was created independently of the body and therefore not necessarily at the time of fertilization. The very early Church favoured the first view, as testified by a number of early Church Councils. But in the Middle Ages it was often thought that animation – the time of the infusion of the human and personal soul – coincided with the completion of foetal formation. Thus the embryo/foetus was not considered to be a person until it was fully formed. And, therefore, the destruction of the early embryo/foetus was not regarded as homicide.

It may be noted that besides the Aristotelian and creationist theories, another influence on Christian discussions about the status of the foetus was the wording of Exodus 21.22–5 in the Septuagint translation, in the third century BC, of the Jewish Bible from Hebrew into Greek. This passage deals with the question of how much compensation should be paid to a husband whose wife has a miscarriage after having been hurt in a fight between two men. In the Hebrew version a miscarriage is to be punished by a fine. No distinction is made between the miscarriage of a formed foetus and the miscarriage of an unformed foetus. But in the Greek version such a distinction is made. Here the death of an unformed foetus is to be punished by a fine, whereas that of a formed foetus is to be punished by 'life for life'. Thus the Greek version suggests that killing a formed foetus is homicide, whereas the killing of an unformed foetus is a lesser crime, a view which came to influence subsequent Christian thought. This was despite the fact that St Jerome's fourth-century Latin version of the text in the Vulgate, the standard Bible in the West, followed the original Hebrew text, which made no distinction between the formed and unformed foetus.

Interestingly, the concept of formation still plays a role in discussions about personhood. For example, a view much like that of Thomas Aquinas is today embraced by some theologians and philosophers who claim that the foetal brain must have reached a certain stage of development before we can speak of a person.[4]

Belonging to another kind of argument in terms of formation are those arguments according to which there can be no embryo proper until a certain stage of embryological development has been reached. These arguments focus on the formation of the growing organism created at fertilization. Their point is not to show when the embryo/foetus acquires a soul or becomes a person. It is to show that we cannot speak of an individual organism, or of individual embryonic life, until some 14 days after fertilization. This is the kind of argument to which we now turn.

THE ARGUMENTS FOR THE 14-DAY LIMIT FOR EMBRYO RESEARCH

It was above all these science-based arguments in terms of embryological development which were the basis for the recommendations made by the Warnock Committee in its report to the UK government.[5] The recommendations made in this Report, then, provided the main rationale for the regulations governing embryo research under the HFE ACT 1990. And the UK law set a trend. Thus it was not only the Warnock Committee that was swayed by this kind of argument; so too were legislators in many other countries. And a number of influential theologians, philosophers and scientists were promoting these arguments worldwide.[6] As a result, it became widely accepted that embryo research is morally justified up until the end of the 14th day after fertilization. However, other European countries took a stand against the creation of embryos expressly for research, whereas the 1990 Act allowed this. Indeed, the European Bioethics Convention of 1997 explicitly banned the creation of embryos for research purposes (Council of Europe, 1997, Article 18.18.2). And so, this Convention was never signed by the UK.

Unlike medieval theologians the aforementioned theologians, philosophers and scientists arguing with reference to embryological development did not however seek an answer to the question: when is the personal soul infused, and so when does personal life begin? Instead they sought an answer to the question: when does individual life begin? This was on the understanding that if the early embryo was not an individual being, then it could not be identified with the later embryo or foetus; and if it could not be so identified it did not deserve our protection. Instead, it was to be seen as a mere disposable aggregate of cells.

The answer to the question posed above at which they arrived was that individual life does not begin until the end of the 14th day after fertilization when the primitive streak appears. This was because only then can we tell whether there will be one individual foetus or two. If there is one primitive streak, there will be one foetus. If there are two primitive streaks, there will be two twin foetuses. And so it was concluded that embryo research was justified up until the appearance of the primitive streak, because only then can we speak of an embryo proper.

To distinguish the 'embryo proper' from the pre-primitive-streak embryo a new term was coined: the pre-primitive-streak embryo was called a pre-embryo. In terms of this new name it was argued, then, that while the embryo proper deserves a degree of respect and protection, the pre-embryo does not. That is to say, it was argued that it is morally justified to undertake research involving the destruction of the pre-embryo. The embryo proper, on the other hand, which deserves a degree of protection, should not be destroyed in research.

FOUR MAIN ARGUMENTS

Four main arguments in terms of embryological development have been advanced to prove that the very early embryo, the so-called pre-embryo, cannot be regarded as an individual organism and therefore cannot be regarded as an embryo proper.

Argument 1

The first argument hangs on the observation that all the cells of the very early embryo are pluri-potent. That is to say, they are undifferentiated: their fate is not yet decided. They have not differentiated into different types of cell, they are still capable of developing into any kind of tissue.[7]

As explained in Chapter 7 of this book, in the context of cloning the reason why an undifferentiated cell has the potential to turn into different kinds of cell is that all (or virtually all) the genes in its nucleus are switched on. By contrast, in a fully differentiated cell, such as a skin cell, only a few genes are switched on. Different genes are switched on in different types of cell. Thus in order for the early embryonic cells to develop into different types of cell, different genes have to be switched off. And this is precisely what happens. Gradually different genes are switched off in different cells, and the cells in the embryo become more and more differentiated. Some become skin cells. Others become neural cells, muscle cells, bone cells and so on.

With reference to these observations, it is concluded that the early embryo cannot be seen as an individual entity. This is because only some of its cells will become the foetus proper. Other cells will develop into extra-embryonic supportive tissue – that is, the amniotic sac, the placenta and the umbilical cord. In other words, it is argued that the entity formed at fertilization is programmed to become not one individual entity but two distinct types of entity. One part of it will become the embryo proper, the first sign of which is the primitive streak. The other part will become the extra-embryonic tissue. And what will become two different types of biological entity cannot be regarded as a single embryo.[8]

Strong counter arguments may, however, be mounted against this line of reasoning. The first is based on the biological observation that the genetic make-up of the placenta and other supportive tissue is the same as that of the embryo/foetus and different from that of the mother. The prenatal test called *chorion villus* sampling is based on this very fact. The test, which was practised already in the 1980s, involves taking a few cells from the chorion, the precursor of the placenta. This is in order to test the genetic health of the foetus. That is to say, this test suggests that the chorion should be counted as a part of the embryonic/foetal organism.

Secondly, the growth of the embryo/foetus is synchronized with that of the extra-embryonic tissue. Noting this, some have argued that the embryo/foetus and the extra-embryonic tissue should be viewed as one organism. The Italian scientist and theologian Antonio Serra spoke of the 'foetus-placenta unit' (Serra, 1988). An American Jesuit theologian, Thomas Daly, argued that the extra-embryonic tissue should be seen as foetal organs, necessary for the organism's intra-uterine development – but no longer needed after birth (Daly, 1987). Thinking on similar lines, Nicholas Tonti-Fillippini, an Australian bioethicist, compared the loss of the placenta at birth to the child's loss of its milk teeth at age six or seven (Tonti-Fillippini, 1987).

Argument 2

According to Argument 2, the early embryo is a mere cluster of cells which, though pluri-potent, may or may not develop successfully into an individual embryo, an embryo proper. This is because cell division after fertilization does not always result in successful embryological development. Things often go wrong. The newly fertilized egg might fail to implant itself in the uterine wall due to a fault in the lining of the womb. Equally, there could be something wrong with the fertilized egg. It might fail to thrive because something went wrong at fertilization. For example, it might be a hydatidiform mole formed by an egg which, having lost its own cell nucleus, is fertilized by two sperm or by a sperm that duplicates itself. Such a product of fertilization is a seriously abnormal entity incapable of developing any foetal tissue. Another type of growth, also incapable of foetal development, is that consisting of a random disorganized mass of foetal tissue.

These observations provide little support for the conclusion that the early embryo is not to be regarded as an individual organism. While it is true that an inhospitable womb may explain failed implantation and a resulting developmental failure of the product of conception, as already noted, the hospitality or inhospitality of the maternal womb tells us nothing about the status of the early embryo. Whether the embryo is an individual entity or not does not depend on the womb. Nor does the abnormality and developmental failure of some products of conception prove that normal products of conception are not individual entities. So this type of argument may be laid to rest.

So too can a simpler, but related, argument. According to a simplified version of Argument 2, put forward already in the 1970s by Bernard Häring (Häring, 1976), the abundant loss of early embryonic life in the case of natural conception, as well as in the case of IVF, tells us that we should not count the early embryo as an embryo proper, or at least not as an individual human being. Some people add that God would not allow the loss of so many nascent human lives. The counter argument here is that the high rate of infant mortality in many parts of the world even today – and in many parts of Europe in the past – does not show us that small children should not be counted as human beings.

Argument 3

Called the twinning argument, Argument 3 is the most convincing argument for saying that individual embryonic life does not start at fertilization. While playing an important role in the debates among scientists in connection with the Warnock report, this argument was mentioned even earlier by a number of theologians and philosophers – themselves, no doubt, influenced by other scientists or medical doctors. Among these theologians were notably Charles Curran (Curran, 1975), Bernard Häring (Häring, 1976) – both Roman Catholic – and Baruch Brody (Brody, 1975), a Jewish scholar.

According to the twinning argument, we cannot speak of an individual embryo, or of individual embryos, until the fertilized egg (the early embryo) has reached the state at which monozygotic twinning is no longer possible (McLaren, 1986). The first one-cell entity formed after fertilization, the fertilized egg, is called a zygote and the word 'mono' means one. Hence, the expression monozygotic twinning, which refers to the division of what started out as one zygote into two new genetically identical embryos. And monozygotic twinning, so it is said, can be observed up until, but not beyond, the 14-day stage and the appearance of the primitive streak. If there is one primitive streak, there is one embryo. If there are two primitive streaks, there are two embryos.[9] This is considered a definitive reason for not thinking of the pre-primitive-streak embryo as an individual organism. Hence, the early embryo is considered a legitimate subject of research.

In brief, the logic behind the twinning argument is the following: monozygotic twinning is the splitting of one biological entity into two organisms. Therefore, there is a discontinuity in the life history of the original entity. The individual lives of monozygotic twins start only at the time of twinning. We should therefore not speak of individual embryonic life until twinning is no longer possible. Nobody knows which zygote will twin.

To counter this powerful argument it might be noted that it is based on the assumption that all newly fertilized embryos have an innate tendency to twin. But this is not true. The majority of embryos never split into two (McLean, 1990). The incidence of monozygotic twinning is a mere 0.36 per cent of live births. This is true for all population groups, which indicates that monozygotic twinning is genetically determined. It also shows that the observation that the early embryo might twin is applicable to a minority of embryos only. That is, the twinning argument is inapplicable with regard to the majority of embryos. Most embryos are continuous individual organisms from the very beginning.

Secondly, monozygotic twinning may be understood as a form of asexual reproduction on a par with budding or the division of an amoeba. Even the plant that propagates by budding is an individual plant. And even the amoeba that has split into two was once a single amoeba, a single life. So why would we not say of an embryo that has split into two that it was an individual embryo before it did so? In addition, the fact that the early embryo might split into two new individual organisms is no reason for according it less respect than the embryo no longer able to twin.

Argument 4

The fourth biological argument for not recognizing the early embryo as an individual organism is based on the lack of spatial orientation of the embryo until the appearance of the primitive streak at the end of the 14th day after fertilization. In other words, it is based on the observation that before the appearance of the primitive streak one cannot tell the top end of the organism from the bottom end. Only when the primitive streak appears can we tell where the head is going to be and where the lower part of the organism is going to be. Moreover, as noted, we know that if there is one primitive streak there is one embryo, and if there are two primitive streaks there are two embryos.

However, the initial organization of the fertilized egg (early embryo) has nothing to do with the entity's individuality. That it is impossible to tell which part of the pre-primitive-streak embryo is to become the head end and which is to become the bottom end does not show that the entity is not an individual organism. Besides, there is growing evidence for the polarity of the embryo from the very beginning. For example, the point at which the sperm enters the egg appears to influence the body-plan of the resulting embryo. The two-cell embryo does not consist of two identical parts, as was previously believed (Piotrowska & Zernick-Goetz, 2001; Poitrowska *et al.*, 2001).

CONCLUSION

We started this chapter with the observation that the rightness or wrongness of deliberately killing the human embryo depends on its moral status. We then outlined the contexts in which human embryos might be deliberately destroyed. It was noted that embryo research might involve embryos left over after IVF as well as embryos created specifically for research. In either case, only pre-14-day embryos are used as a result of the scientific debates preceding the UK legislation, which set a trend worldwide.

Having noted that the environment of the embryo does not impact on its moral status, and having given a cursory look at ancient views on embryological development and animation, we turned in the second part of this chapter to four main arguments proposed by scientists for not regarding the pre-14-day embryo as an individual being – even if clearly it is a human being, since it is a living organism of human origin.

We found that the weightiest of these arguments was the twinning argument. And, not surprisingly, it was the twinning argument coupled with the observation that the primitive streak is an important biological landmark that was the most influential in the debates preceding the UK legislation regulating embryo research (Warnock, 1984: 65).

Of all four arguments, only the twinning argument tells us something about the individuality of the embryo. But while it tells us that some embryos only begin their individual existence some time after fertilization when twinning takes place, it is not a convincing argument for saying that the very early embryo deserves less respect than the post-14-day embryo no longer capable of twinning.

As to the term pre-embryo mentioned above, it did initially play an important role in the debates deciding the fate of many embryos created *in vitro*. But it was a short-lived term. Nowhere was it used in the HFE Act 1990. One reason why the term is no longer fashionable is the recognition that the development of the embryo is a gradual process starting at fertilization.[10] No stage marks a radically new beginning in this gradual process starting at fertilization, except at the time of twinning. And even when the embryo twins, the different developmental stages follow one another in the same ordered succession.

Finally, for many debating the status of the human embryo and foetus the most interesting question is not whether the early embryo is an individual being but whether it is a person. And personhood is often linked to the possession of certain abilities. As we have seen, Aristotle and Aquinas linked the personal soul, that is, the rational soul, to the physiological structures of the foetus required to house a rational soul and enable it to exercise its rational capacities. Today a similar line of argument is taken up by those who argue that in order to be a person it is necessary to be self-conscious and have the ability to reason. There is, however, a noteworthy difference between them and Aristotle and Aquinas. On the views of Aristotle and Aquinas, it is sufficient to have the potential to exercise intellectual abilities in order to be counted as a person. By contrast, some present-day philosophers argue that it is necessary to be able actually to exercise intellectual abilities in order to be counted as a person. And because not all human beings are capable of so doing, they argue that not all human beings are persons.

It is to the question of the validity of this kind of argument which excludes many humans that we turn in the next chapter.

CHAPTER 3

RESPECT FOR HUMAN LIFE AND PERSONHOOD

This being premised, to find wherein personal identity consists, we must consider what person stands for: which I think, is a thinking intelligent being, that has reason and reflection, and can consider itself as itself, the same thinking thing in different times and places; which it does only by that consciousness which is inseparable from thinking, and, as it seems to me, essential to it: it being impossible for anyone to perceive without perceiving that he does perceive.

John Locke (Locke, 2004: 302)

INTRODUCTION: THE LOCKEAN VIEW

It was in book 2, chapter 27, in the second edition of his *Essay Concerning Human Understanding*, published in 1694, that John Locke (1632–1704) put forward his famous definition of a person as a self-conscious, thinking and intelligent being. This understanding of personhood in terms of intellectual abilities and self-consciousness has set its stamp on much subsequent discussion of the question: what does it mean to be a person?

In this chapter we shall examine and compare the merits of the Lockean and a number of other understandings of personhood. The question of who is or is not a person is important for many decisions in the field of medical ethics. Persons, and in particular competent persons, are accorded special rights. Locke's definition homes in on self-consciousness. This is, of course, a typical characteristic of a sane and healthy mature person. But is self-consciousness the most important characteristic of a person?

Locke made a distinction between 'man' and 'person'. This distinction is adopted by several contemporary philosophers influential in the field of bioethics. Like Locke, they do not equate persons with human beings. To their mind, as to Locke's, the distinguishing mark of a person is self-consciousness, entailing an awareness of one's own past and a concern for one's future. Locke wrote: 'This personality [person] extends itself beyond present existence to what is past, only by consciousness, whereby it becomes concerned and accountable, owns and imputes to itself past actions. . .' (Locke, 2004: 312).

But not all human beings are self-conscious and aware of their past and of the future. And so, on a Lockean understanding, the permanently comatose human being is no longer a person, nor is the infant. Just how sharply Locke distinguished between the concept of a person and that of a man, or a human being, is shown by the following passage: 'For should the soul of a prince, carrying with it the consciousness of the prince's past life, enter and inform the body of a cobbler, as soon as deserted by its own soul, everyone sees he would be the same person with the prince, accountable only for the prince's actions; but who would say it was the same man? The body . . . would, I guess, to everybody determine the man in this case . . .' (Locke, 2004: 306). The passage shows that while Locke identified the man (the human being) with the material body, he identified the person with the self-conscious mind.

An equally sharp separation between body and mind was made by the French philosopher Rene Descartes (1596–1650), born some 40 years before Locke. In his *Meditations*, he too identified the person with the thinking self-conscious mind. On this kind of dualist understanding, the person is a non-spatial entity, while the body becomes mere spatial material.

Another influential thinker who should be mentioned is the eighteenth-century German philosopher Immanuel Kant. His understanding of a person is similar to that of Locke and Descartes inasmuch as it homes in on the rationality of agents. Indeed, to Kant's mind, rationality is the criterion of personhood. In his *Groundwork of the Metaphysics of Morals* he said of 'rational beings' that they 'are called persons because their nature already marks them out as ends in themselves – that is, as something which ought not to be used merely as means' (Kant, 1998: 66). For him, rational agents alone belong to the realm of morality, for they alone are ends in themselves. On Kant's account, not only are persons identified with reference to their rationality, but, in addition, they have a special moral status wherefore they are worthy of special respect. And so he argued that you should 'act in such a way that you always treat humanity [human persons] whether in your own person or in the person of any other, never simply as a means, but always at the same time as an end' (Kant, 1998: 66).

Locke and Descartes as well as Kant, then, identified persons in terms of mental attributes and, in particular, rational attributes. Their criteria of personhood therefore exclude many members of the human family. On elitist and intellectualist understandings such as theirs, which ascribe personhood only to those actually in possession of certain mental functions or capacities such as self-consciousness and rationality, neither those human beings who have not yet developed the mental characteristics typical of sound and mature persons, nor those who have lost these characteristics, can be counted as persons. On elitist understandings such as these, neither the human embryo, nor the foetus, nor the infant can be counted as persons. Equally, personhood is denied to the severely brain damaged and to the senile old lady who no longer recognizes her relatives.

On the other hand, there would be no question of denying the humanity of the brain damaged or the senile old lady. Their bodies, like that of Locke's cobbler, are clearly human. This is also true of the infant as well as of the fully formed foetus. For they too have bodies that are easily identifiable as human. The situation is more problematic for the human embryo not yet in possession of a recognizably human body.

However, exclusive understandings of the Lockean type, which distinguish between persons and human, are clearly counter-intuitive. We do count infants and senile old ladies as persons (at least many of us do). Mostly we do not distinguish between humans and persons, though sometimes we do. God may be said to be a person. Indeed, on a Christian Trinitarian understanding, God comprises three persons: the Father, the Son and the Holy Spirit. But leaving God aside – as well as angels – we usually use the words 'human being' and 'person' interchangeably, even if it may sound a bit odd to describe the newly conceived embryo as a person, although, *pace* the scientific arguments discussed in Chapter 2, it is indisputably a human being. Yet, retrospectively we might speak of John or Joanna when referring to them as newly conceived, and this raises the question whether or not we should use the term 'person' inclusively and apply it to all humans.

The last question is important. It is important because our understanding of what it means to be a person determines our attitudes to embryos, foetuses and infants as well as to those human beings who have lost or have never fully developed the mental faculties typical of hale and healthy adults. How we treat these groups of human beings depends on whether we consider them to be persons. If we see them as persons, we cannot treat them as disposable material to be used in research or say that their lives are not worth living. By contrast, if we see the embryo as a non-person its destruction will not worry us and we might say, as some present-day philosophers do, that some lives are not worth living.

PETER SINGER'S UNDERSTANDING OF PERSONHOOD

Arguing on Lockean lines, the Princeton philosopher Peter Singer adopts as sole criterion of personhood the actual possession of certain mental abilities, among them self-consciousness and a degree of rationality. For this reason he does not count all members of the human family as persons. So who does he count as a person?

> In the Netherlands, a few years ago, an observer reported on the lives of some people confined in a new kind of institution. These people had a special condition that did not handicap them at all physically, but intellectually they were well below the normal human level; they could not speak, although they made noises and gestures . . . They rarely spent time alone, and they appeared to have no difficulty in understanding each other's gestures and vocalisations . . .
>
> Although monogamy was not practised, the leader tried to prevent others having sex with his favourites. To get around this, flirtations leading up to sexual intercourse were conducted with a good deal of discretion, so as not to attract the leader's attention.
>
> (Singer, 1995a: 159–61)

The quotation is from Singer's book *Rethinking Life and Death*. Having provided this account of the life of the inmates in an institution in the Dutch town of Arnhem, he writes: 'I have described this community in some detail because I want to raise an ethical question about the way in which people with this condition were regarded by those who looked after them. In the eyes of the supervisors the inmates did not have the same kind of right to life as normal human beings' (Singer, 1995a: 161–2).

According to Singer, the inmates were not treated with the respect due to them. Surely, he is right! Should not all people be treated with the same respect? Well, perhaps the reader has already guessed that the people Singer is talking about are not human beings. They are chimpanzees.

While the kind of creature to which the term 'person' normally refers is human, Singer argues that the term is applicable also to the apes, that is, chimpanzees, gorillas and orang-utans. This is because of their advanced intellectual abilities. To his mind, an animal should be regarded as a person if it possesses rationality and self-consciousness and has the ability to plan for the future and look back at the past.

Because Singer regards the apes as persons, he also argues that they have certain rights, such as the right to be treated better than the inmates in the Arnhem institution. In other words, he feels that we should show more respect for chimpanzees. In his view, the attitude of the zoo-keepers in Arnhem was an expression of 'speciesism'. Those who are 'specist' give preferential treatment to members of their own species: they see members of their own species as superior to members of other species.

Of course, Singer is right when he says that most of us humans are 'specist'. In particular, those of us who identify ourselves with the Judaeo-Christian tradition of thought are unabashedly 'specist', for on the Christian understanding, human beings are thought to have a unique relationship with God inasmuch as we are created in his image and are appointed his stewards of creation. No other kind of creature is thought to have moral responsibilities, since humans alone are capable of self-consciously responding to God, by seeking to do his work – or turning their back on him. This is why, according to Christian teaching, humans have a special dignity and why human life has a special value.

That said, Christians are not alone in thinking that humans are special. Indeed, most humans are specist. And this is with good reason. Are we not as a species more intelligent than other species? Surely only humans have moral responsibilities? So surely we are superior to other animals? Disagreeing with this kind reasoning, Singer has little time for this view of humankind. He does not think that membership of the species *Homo sapiens* gives the individual a special status and dignity that makes certain claims on us. He argues that the worth of human life varies and that 'life without consciousness is of no worth at all' (Singer, 1995a: 190). To him the ethically relevant characteristics of a creature, and those in virtue of which it is a person, are the actual possession of mental characteristics and abilities such as consciousness, self-consciousness and rationality.[1] Those humans who do not yet have, never will have, or have lost these kinds of intellectual powers or characteristics, have no right to special respect, and have less right to life than a mature and mentally healthy gorilla. To quote Singer:

> Membership of the species *Homo sapiens* is not ethically relevant, any characteristic or combination of characteristics that we regard as giving human beings a right to life or as making it generally wrong to end a human life, may be possessed by some nonhuman animals. If they are, then we must grant those nonhuman animals the same right to life as we grant to human beings . . .
> (Singer, 1995a: 205)

According to Singer, then, human foetuses and babies are not persons because they are not self-conscious and rational. Thus, he and his colleague, Helga Kuhse, have suggested that 'a period of twenty-eight days after birth might be allowed before an infant is accepted as having the same right to life as others' (Singer, 1995a: 217; Kuhse and Singer, 1985: 194). It follows on the same line of reasoning that the senile and disoriented old lady who can no longer recognize her relatives is not a person either. In Singer's view, we should not speak of a person unless we have before us someone who is actually capable of manifesting personal intellectual abilities.

If most of us are specist, Singer is elitist. Holding that life is of little or no value without the possession of certain intellectual abilities, he does not give preferential treatment to humans as such, but he does give preferential treatment to those humans and other creatures who are in possession of certain mental characteristics. But is this in keeping with common sense?

A PERSON IS A BODILY INDIVIDUAL WITH A RATIONAL NATURE

The word 'person' is derived from the Latin word 'persona', which referred to the actor's mask in classical drama. The 'persona' was a character-mask. It was associated with different types of character and roles. Used, then, to refer to a character or to certain characteristics, the word 'persona' was not unlike the Lockean term 'person'. Both terms point to certain personal characteristics, without necessarily linking them to a particular body.

The term person was later also used in Christian discussions about the concept of the Trinity as defined in outline at the Councils of Nicaea (325) and Constantinople (381) and dogmatized at that of Chalcedon (451). According to the Trinitarian understanding of God, the One God exists in one substance and three persons, Father, Son and Holy Spirit. And this understanding is said to be a mystery neither knowable without revelation nor provable in the light of it.

Leaving the Trinity aside, a more helpful definition for our understanding of ordinary human personhood was that proposed by a Christian thinker, Boethius (*c*. 480–524). He defined a person as: 'an individual substance of a rational nature' (Boethius, 1891: 1342 sqq). It should be noted that according to the Boethian definition of a person, which influenced among others Thomas Aquinas (Aquinas, ST I qq 21, 29), the substance and its nature are inseparable. The term person points at once in two directions. It points to a unique individual substance, which insofar as it is mortal is physical and so has a history. At the same time it indicates the nature of this substance. Thus, on the Boethian definition a person is a unique individual being with a life history and with a certain nature, that is, a rational nature.

If Locke's understanding was dualistic and separated body and mind, here we have a holistic understanding. Based on this holistic understanding, is the well rehearsed argument from potentiality, according to which the human embryo has the potential to become an individual with the intellectual characteristics typical of sane and healthy adult human beings.

THE ARGUMENT FROM POTENTIALITY

Let us consider, then, the situation of those human beings, such as embryos, foetuses and newborn infants, who are not yet self-conscious and rational, who do not yet possess the intellectual abilities typical of the archetypal group of persons, namely sane and mature human adults. What they have is a genetic make-up that makes them human. Moreover, this genetic make-up carries with it certain potentialities, or certain capacities. In virtue of their genetic make-up they are oriented to become human beings with the intellectual characteristics typical of sane and mature adult persons. That is to say, provided there is no programme error in their genetic make-up, and provided nothing goes wrong with their development, and provided they are not destroyed on purpose, they will become human adults with typically human intellectual abilities. Inbuilt in the normal embryonic human individual is an original potential, or capacity, to become a human person with the intellectual abilities typical of adult members of the human species.

The embryo's genetic make-up may be understood as a plan. The genetic make-up directs the development of the embryo. The development of the embryo of every species is goal-directed. A (normal) cat embryo is programmed to become an adult cat. A (normal) human embryo is programmed to become a human adult. The genes contain the information required for the embryo's development. If all goes well, the human embryo will increasingly realize its potential to develop the characteristics typical of healthy human adults. The potential to develop normal human and personal intellectual abilities is there within the (normal) human embryo from the very beginning. In other words, a (normal) human embryo is a person, in the making.

This was noted already by Tertullian, a staunch defender of the Christian Church against accusations that its members practised homicide and infanticide. In the *Apologia* he argued that the acorn should already be regarded as an oak. Similarly, he argued that a human person in the making must already be seen as a human person – and so to kill it is homicide: 'It makes no difference whether you snatch away the soul after birth or destroy it while coming to birth. Even the man who is yet to be is a man; just as every fruit is already present in the seed' (Tertullian, 1997a: 9.8). On this understanding, whatever has the potential to become a mature human person is already a human person. It is not just a potential person, it is a person with potential.

The human embryo is not yet self-conscious, nor yet capable of reasoning or planning for the future or looking back at its past, but provided it is healthy and is neither intentionally destroyed nor the victim of an accident, it will develop these abilities over time. Already from the start, it has within itself the capacity to acquire the intellectual abilities typical of an adult human being, a person.

The human adult's self-consciousness and ability to reason, plan for the future and look back at the past do not come from nowhere, they come from its human nature (Iglesias, 1987: 35; Sutton, 1990: 116).

Indeed, we might say that the human embryo's potential to develop typically personal characteristics comes from its personal nature. This would seem to be the position of the Roman Catholic Church's Congregation for the Doctrine of the Faith. In its document *Donum Vitae* of 1987, it argued that 'the conclusions of science regarding the human embryo provide a valuable indication for discerning by the use of reason a personal presence at the moment of its first appearance of human life' (Congregation for the Doctrine of the Faith, 1987, Part I, para. 1).

Two American Dominican theologians, Benedict Ashley and Kevin O'Rourke, adopt a similar understanding. This is one that looks both to the past and to the future. They say that a human subject should be counted as a person not only if it has in itself the capacity to become a person, but also if it once possessed, but now has lost, the intellectual capacities typical of persons. They argue that even if the definition of personhood centres around the intellectual abilities typical of sane and healthy humans, the term person should be used to apply to 'the entire biography of the unique organism . . . not only actual, here and now performance must be taken into account' (Ashley and O'Rourke, 1989: 209–10). In other words, on this holistic and historical understanding of personhood – according to which human and personal life is seen as a whole from the time of birth, or conception, to the time of death – whoever will be or has been a mature person, with the intellectual abilities typical of a person, should be counted as a person. This is entirely reasonable. Most of us actually count as persons both the infant and the very senile and disoriented old person with memory loss. Many of us even name the foetus in the womb, especially now that ultrasound allows parents to take home a photograph of their recognizably human 12-week-old foetus.

However, the argument from potentiality, like that with reference to the entire life-history of the individual, arguably leaves open the question of the status of those unfortunate members of the human species who, for some reason, never develop to the full the intellectual abilities belonging to the archetypal person. What, if any, are the reasons for counting them as persons?

THE *IMAGO DEI* AND THE FAMILIAL UNDERSTANDINGS OF PERSONHOOD

The Christian answer to the question above is: each one of us humans is created in the *Imago Dei*. As already noted, on the Genesis account in the Bible, the human being as such is afforded a special status and dignity on account of being created in the image of God: 'So God created man in his own image, in the image of God he created him; male and female he created them' (Gen. 1.27). Only human beings are spoken of in this manner. On the biblical understanding, not only were the very first humans, Adam and Eve, created in the image of God, but all their descendants are created in the image of God. In Genesis 5, Adam is said to have 'fathered a son in his own likeness, after his image' (Gen. 5.3). His son, then, must also be in the image of God, as must the son of his son.

The Genesis stories may be allegorical, but they contain a lot of wisdom when singling out human beings as special. Most of us do, and for good reason. For a start, not only are we, as a species, more intelligent than animals, but, as argued above, we are the only creatures to which we ascribe moral responsibility. Humans are the only kind of creature we hold morally accountable for their actions. Secondly, the Genesis stories speak of the human family as one and of the child as being in this image of its parents. This is with the implication that the child shares their nature; and so, since its parents are persons, the child too is a person.

When the emphasis is put on the familial dimension of personhood, no human being can be excluded from the human family, the family of human persons. Being born of woman immediately places one within the human family and in a personal relationship with other persons. On this understanding every child born to human parents counts as a person. Being of human origin means being a member of the wider human community of persons; the ability or disability of the child is irrelevant. Being of human origin, it is human; and being human it is a person.

On this familial, relational and inclusive understanding, it makes no difference whether, because of accident and injury or illness, the human being does not manifest those intellectual abilities or mental characteristics we associate with personhood. The human person is identified as such because of his or her human, and thus personal, nature and his or her familial relationship with other persons.

CONCLUSION

Having examined Lockean understandings of personhood and found them wanting, we turned to more inclusive understandings. Unlike the intellectualist and elitist understandings of a Locke or Singer, these more inclusive ideas we found more in keeping with common sense and intuition. While the argument from potentiality accommodates infants as well as more mature individuals, the understanding on which human life must be seen as whole from its beginning to the end includes not only infants but also very old people who may have lost their memory or other personal abilities. The most inclusive understanding, and one that fits in well with everyday thinking, is that on which every human child is counted as a person, simply because it is a member of the human family. On this understanding, everyone of human origin is counted as a person, even if he or she does not actually manifest the intellectual abilities typical of sane and healthy adult members of our species.

The Lockean type of understanding remains, however, influential, as is shown in the following chapters. It is on the basis of this type of elitist understanding, coupled with other dominant philosophies such as utilitarianism and Darwinism, that much of the debates about abortion and euthanasia, as well as those about genetic testing and gene therapy, are implicitly, if not explicitly, couched. The intellectually able and able-bodied are given preferential consideration. The lives of those lacking in mental or physical health or social utility are considered to be of lesser value. And some lives are considered not worth living.

Quality of life is, of course, important: mental and physical health is a blessing. But the question is whether some persons are lesser beings and whether their lives are of less value than others, or whether human life is of intrinsic value? The answer to this question is important for medical decision-making and social policies.

In the next chapter the ethos of a 'new medicine' will be pitched against the traditional Hippocratic and Christian ethos. It will be shown that, unlike the Christian and Hippocratic tradition of medicine, this new medicine does not accord intrinsic value to every human life.

CHAPTER 4

ABORTION: QUALITY *VERSUS* SANCTITY OF LIFE

And I will use regiments for the benefit of the ill in accordance with my ability and my judgement, but from [what is] to their harm or injustice I will keep [them]. And I will not give a drug that is deadly to anyone if asked [for it], nor will I suggest the way to such counsel. And likewise I will not give a woman a destructive pessary [i.e., procure an abortion].

Hippocratic Oath, *c.* 400 BC (Miles, 2004: xiii–xiv)

INTRODUCTION: QUALITY *VERSUS* SANCTITY OF LIFE

Dating from about 400 BC, the Hippocratic Oath presents a view of the medical profession as a healing profession opposed to the taking of life. Rediscovered in the Middle Ages it was adapted to Christian thought, as it sat well with a Christian ethics. And from the eighteenth century onwards various versions of the oath were widely used in graduation ceremonies in European and American medical schools. Even today many European and American medical schools incorporate some kind of oath into their graduation ceremonies, though these oaths tend to be coloured by secular influences. The increasing secularization of Western society means that the traditional Christian understanding of the sanctity and dignity of human life is being challenged by other visions.

Coupled with the development of new diagnostic techniques and technically advanced ways of sustaining life, the secularization of our society has promoted a new medical ethics. According to this new ethics, the value of human life is measured in terms of its quality, that is, in terms of the physical and mental health and well-being of the patient. A concept of quality of life has been pitched against the principle of the sanctity of life and so against the Christian understanding of the intrinsic dignity and value of every human life. Today, then, the medical tradition emphasizing the principle of the sanctity of human life is competing with another school of thought according to which some lives are not worth living, because they are perceived to be of too poor a quality.

The new medicine is coloured by Lockean, Kantian and utilitarian influences. The Lockean influence is evident inasmuch as some humans are not afforded a proper personal status because they lack certain mental abilities. The utilitarian influence comes to the fore above all in an emphasis on happiness and wellbeing, while a strong emphasis on patient autonomy reflects a Kantian influence.

Of course, there is nothing wrong with the utilitarian aim to promote wellbeing or happiness and avoid causing pain and suffering. That is, there is nothing wrong with this, provided it does not entail a devaluation of some lives because of poor quality or lack of certain talents. But if it does, then some members of the human family may be at risk. Their lives may be seen as dispensable and the interests of others or of society may take priority.

There is nothing wrong with respect for patient autonomy either, unless it means that doctors should act as shopkeepers ever ready to meet customer demands. As the American bioethicist, and former chair of the President's Council on Bioethics, Leon Kass has pointed out, the traditional end of medicine is not one of satisfying the patient's more or less rational wishes but one of healing or alleviating suffering, though never by killing the patient. Acts primarily aimed at satisfying patients' desires are, he says, 'acts not of medicine but of indulgence or gratification' (Kass, 1985: 159).[1]

While measuring the value of life on different scales, what the old and the new medicine have in common is a claim to compassion. Both seek to alleviate human suffering. The old tradition is no less sensitive to pain and suffering than the new medicine; like the new medicine, it seeks to promote quality of life, but while the new medicine is prepared to shorten some lives in order to avoid pain and suffering, bioethicists and practitioners adhering to the old sanctity-of-life tradition will not allow the deliberate killing of the sick even for the sake of alleviating his suffering.

On the other hand, if there is a question of life against life, even bioethicists and doctors in the old tradition might allow one life to be sacrificed to save the other. Abortion in order to save the mother's life is a case of this kind. Another case of life against life is that of Siamese twins unable to survive together, while one of them might survive if they were separated.

In this chapter and the next we will explore the difference between the old and the new medicine. In this chapter we will do so with focus on abortion and in the next chapter with focus on euthanasia. Thus we will start this chapter with a brief comparison between the new so-called four principles approach, and the traditional approach espoused by the twentieth-century theologian Karl Barth, as well as by John Paul II in the encyclical letter *Evangelium Vitae*. We will then examine the Christian tradition with respect to abortion and look at current abortion law and reasons for and against abortion.

FOUR ACCLAIMED PRINCIPLES *VERSUS* THE TRADITIONAL CHRISTIAN AND HIPPOCRATIC APPROACH

Seeking to present a medical ethics suited to twentieth-century medicine, the American bioethicists Tom Beauchamp and James Childress produced what is now regarded as a classical work in medical ethics. While retaining the Hippocratic principle not to harm the patient, they reinterpreted it in such a way as to accommodate a quality-of-life ethics. Their work, entitled *Principles of Biomedical Ethics*, was first published in 1979 and has since gone through several editions. In it the authors specify four principles of medical ethics: respect for the patient's autonomy; nonmaleficence (doing no harm); beneficence and justice.

The first principle, that of autonomy, is one to which it is hard to take exception, except when it is used to prioritize patient demands over the proper ends of medical practice. With reference to Kant's respect for autonomous agents and Mill's insistence on respecting individual rights without inflicting harm on others, the authors tell us that the desires of those who have 'the capacity to determine their own destiny' should be respected, unless doing so would harm other people (Beauchamp and Childress, 2001: 64). This principle is important, of course, insofar as it means that, with the exception of minors or other incompetent patients, the patient must have given his or her informed consent before being subjected to a medical procedure. Equally, it is important insofar as it means that in the case of an incompetent patient a guardian or attorney must give consent on the patient's behalf (Beauchamp and Childress, 2001: 57–112).

The emphasis on consent rightly ensures respect for the patient's own understanding, or that of his guardian, of what is in his or her best interest. It is unreasonable, however, to demand that doctors do things that are against their conscience or contrary to professional standards or the law.

Coupled with the second principle – not to harm the patient – the first principle, however, may be used to support practises that once formed no part of medical practice. Together with the first principle, the second principle not to harm the patient is therefore controversial. Spelled out in such a way that it does not exclude helping a patient to die by physician-assisted suicide, it supports practices that are at odds with the old medicine, most legislations and widely accepted mores. The following quotation mentions a doctor, Quill, who prescribed barbiturates to a patient suffering from leukaemia: 'Suffering and loss of cognitive capacity can ravage and dehumanise patients so severely that death is in their best interests. In these tragic situations, physicians like Quill do not act wrongly in assisting competent patients to bring about their deaths' (Beauchamp and Childress, 2001: 151).

So, to the mind of Beauchamp and Childress, assisted suicide – and possibly even the active killing of a patient at his or her request – is not necessarily a harmful act. Rather, as an act that respects the wishes of the patient and alleviates suffering, it may be seen as a gesture of compassion. The medical ethics espoused by Beauchamp and Childress is a clear example, then, of a quality-of-life ethics, as opposed to a sanctity-of-life ethics.

As to the principle of beneficence, it comes in two forms. As a patient-centred principle, its focus is on the good of the individual patient. Action in line with this principle might take the form of paternalism and clash with the first principle. But while the two authors may hold that a certain amount of paternalism could be justified in some cases, in line with a general trend, they prioritize the first principle. Paternalism is no longer welcome, especially as many patients today are well informed not least thanks to the internet. In its second form the principle of benevolence serves to help doctors weigh up costs and benefits of using, for example, certain drugs to treat certain kinds of illness. Here the cost and benefits are not to individual patients but to types of patient or to institutions or society at large (Beauchamp and Childress, 2001: 165–224).

As to the fourth principle, that of justice, the authors argue for everyone's right to a decent minimum level of health care. Their argument is very much reliant on the American model of insurance-based healthcare, and it raises the question of what constitutes a decent minimum. The authors do discuss the British, Scandinavian and Canadian systems of providing free health care at the point of use for all, but doubt that such systems could be implemented everywhere. They suggest, however, that these systems are fairer than the American system which involves considerable inequality in access to services (Beauchamp and Childress, 2001: 272).

It is, as argued, the second of these four principles which, when coupled with the first, reveals a clear shift away from the traditional Christian and Hippocratic medical ethics. Today this shift away from traditional medical ethics has many influential sympathizers. The most well-known proponent of a medical ethics with emphasis on quality of life, Peter Singer, voices a fierce attack on advocates of the principle of sanctity of human life. Not surprisingly, he is especially scathing of the medical ethics of the Roman Catholic Church. In his book *Rethinking Life and Death*, Singer proposes five new commandments, the joint message of which is that not all lives are of equal value and that some lives are not worth living. In other words, hampered by mental or physical illness or disability, some human lives are better cut short by abortion or euthanasia.

The British bioethicist John Harris takes the same view: 'There can surely be no doubt that killing such who want to die, for whom death is the best prospect, and who cannot kill themselves, is not only the right moral choice but also a caring and humane thing to do' (Harris, 1985: 78). However, as observed by the Christian bioethicist Gilbert Meilaender, on a Christian view of life and death, euthanasia is never acceptable: 'In the Christian world, in which death and suffering are great evils but not the greatest evil, love can never include in its meaning hastening a fellow human being toward (the evil of) death, nor can it mean a refusal to acknowledge death when it comes (as an evil but not the greatest evil)' (Meilaender, 1989: 458).

Thus the Reformist twentieth-century theologian Karl Barth describes euthanasia as 'a type of killing which can be regarded only as murder, i.e., as wicked usurpation of God's sovereign right over life and death' (Barth, 1966: 422). And needless to say, the Roman Catholic view as voiced by John Paul II in *Evangelium Vitae* could not be further removed from those of Singer and Harris. For him life is always a good, as is clear from the following passage:

Life is always a good. Why is life a good? This question is found everywhere in the Bible. And from the very first pages it receives a powerful and amazing answer. The life which God gives man is quite different from the life of all other living creatures, inasmuch as man, although formed from the dust of the earth (cf. Gn 2:7; 3:19; Job 34:15; Ps 103:14, 104:29) is a manifestation of God in the world, a sign of His presence, a trace of His glory (cf. Gn 1:26–27; Ps 8:6). (John Paul II, 1995, para. 34)

Not only does John Paul II describe human life as a special good because it is a gift from God and in his image, but he does so also because he sees it as a pilgrimage 'to its final end, to its destiny of fellowship with God in knowledge and love of Him' (John Paul II, 1995, para. 38). On a Christian understanding, then, human life has an intrinsic value both because of its origin and because of its final end. And on this understanding of life as an intrinsic good, it is hard to defend the taking of human life. In other words, this understanding is supportive of the traditional Hippocratic medical ethics that will not allow doctors to take human life.

ABORTION AND CONTRACEPTION IN TIMES PAST

Abortion is no novelty, and early abortion has generally been seen as a lesser evil than late abortion. While in the Middle Ages this had much to do with beliefs about the moral status of the foetus, since early times it has been well recognized that early abortion is less dangerous for the woman. The dangers of surgical abortion were also well recognized. Thus, because of the dangers involved, surgical methods were not much in use in ancient times. Most ancient literature on the subject of abortion therefore speaks about vaginal suppositories or oral abortifacients, and it is noteworthy that the Hippocratic Oath condemned the use of the knife for any reason, in addition to forbidding the use of poisons or suppositories to induce abortion (Riddle, 1994: 7). Actually, in Graeco-Roman antiquity surgical operations were the prerogative of barbers.

It should also be recognized that the distinction between abortifacients and contraceptives has been understood since times immemorial, and it was well known among the ancients that some suppositories and oral drugs might work both as contraceptives and as abortifacients – just like the so-called morning-after pill used today. Dioscorides (*c.* 40–90), the first-century Greek physician and author of *De Materia Medica*, the precursor of modern pharmacopaedias, knew of a number of contraceptive drugs, many of which also worked as abortifacients. So too did Soranus (*c.* 98–138), a second-century Greek physician practising in Rome and antiquity's best-known writer on gynaecological issues (Riddle, 1995: 25–6). Not surprisingly, the early Church condemned both contraceptives and abortifacients as anti-life and contrary to divine intentions.

Even today the Roman Catholic Church condemns both contraception and abortion. According to canon law, women who have an abortion, and anyone who helps them, automatically excommunicate themselves; and no distinction is made between early and late abortion. While condemned in Paul VI's encyclical *Humanae Vitae* of 1968, contraception is, however, regarded as a lesser sin not warranting excommunication. Indeed, Paul VI's condemnation of contraception has been very controversial within the Roman Catholic Church and widely disregarded by the faithful.

If we look back at the history of the Church's views on abortion, we find, however, that it has varied. The early church councils made no distinction between early and late abortion. As far as we know, the Irish Penitentials of 675 were the first to differentiate between early and late abortion (Jones, 2004: 67–8; Sutton, 1990: 181–2). But at the time there was no universal practice. At the Council of Worms (848), abortion at any stage was condemned as homicide, and it would appear that during the next few centuries often no distinction was made between early and late abortion. But in the eleventh century the distinction was taken up again by Ivo, Bishop of Chartres, in his *Decretum*, and in the twelfth century it was confirmed by Gratian in his collection *Decretum Gratiani*, and also by Peter Lombard in his *Sentences*. However, since neither of these works had the status of canon law (Jones, 2004: 69–72; Sutton, 1990: 183–4), it fell on Pope Innocent III to incorporate the distinction in church legislation. This was by means of papal letter, *Sicut et Literrarum*, written around 1220. But even after this there was no uniform penitential practice until 1591, when Pope Gregory XIV instituted excommunication for abortion of the formed foetus only (Jones, 2004: 72). His ruling remained decisive, however, until 1869 when Pope Pius IX abolished the distinction between early and late abortion in the light of medical evidence showing that there was no sharp physiological distinction between the early and the late foetus.

And so the ruling that a woman who has an abortion automatically excommunicates herself dates from this time.

Another interesting development within church legislation relates to arguments put forward in the fourteenth and fifteenth centuries in favour of abortion in order to save the mother's life. One of these arguments failed to convince the Roman Catholic Church; the other succeeded. The one that failed was produced by the fourteenth-century Dominican, St Antoninus, Archbishop of Florence (1389–1459), who in citing another Dominican, John of Naples, argued that it was not a sin to destroy an unanimated foetus in order to save the mother's life (Jones, 2004: 178–9; Sutton, 1990: 185).

What did gain magisterial approval was the argument in terms of the principle of double-effect. This argument was produced by the Franciscan theologian Antonius Corduba (1485–1578). It had nothing to do with the soul of the foetus or with its formation. Instead Corduba argued that it was permissible indirectly to kill the foetus as an unintended side-effect of saving the mother (see Jones, 2004: 179; Sutton, 1990: 185–6). It is noteworthy that this kind of reasoning is still used by Christian doctors who do not accept abortion. It serves to justify the removal of a cancerous uterus to save a pregnant woman's life, even if it has the side-effect of killing the unborn child. It is also applicable in the case of an ectopic pregnancy when in order to save the life of the mother it is necessary to remove the fallopian tube containing the foetus. In these situations it is argued that the good of the intended act of saving the mother outweighs the unfortunate but unintended death of the foetus.

ABORTION AND THE LAW

In most countries abortion was an illegal practice well into the last century. It was not until 1938 that the first steps were taken to liberalize the abortion law in Great Britain so as to allow abortion not merely to preserve the mother's life, but also to preserve her physical and mental health. With the Abortion Act of 1967, applicable in England, Wales and Scotland, but not in Northern Ireland, the reasons for abortion were further extended. Thus the 1967 Act allowed abortion up to 28 weeks' gestation for the sake of the physical or mental health of the woman and any existing children in her family, as well as when there was a substantial risk that the child would suffer from serious mental or physical abnormalities (Abortion

Act 1967, section 1 (1)). But since the 28-week limit was chosen on the ground that the foetus was thought viable outside the maternal womb at that stage, after the 28th week abortion was not allowed except in order to save the woman's life.

If many of the arguments preceding the Act centred on the need to legalize abortion in order to avoid backstreet abortion and the risk of maternal death, the law of 1967 was also a reflection of new more liberal sexual mores in the 1960s and a greater emphasis on women's rights. Thus the UK was not the only country to introduce a liberal abortion policy at that time; most other European countries witnessed similar developments in the 1960s and 1970s. Portugal and Ireland were exceptions. Portugal only recently legalized abortion, whereas in Ireland it remains illegal. In the USA with a constitution emphasizing individual rights, abortion was legalized in 1971 as a result of the famous Roe v. Wade case, in which the United States Supreme Court ruled that American state laws forbidding abortion violated the US constitutional right to privacy.

Today, then, the unborn child no longer enjoys the protection it had while the Hippocratic ethic reigned in medicine and was recognized in law. Its interests are now explicitly rated second to that of the mother and her family. Thus, in *The Declaration of Oslo: Statement on Therapeutic Abortion*, the World Medical Association states that, given the 'diversity of attitudes towards the life of the unborn child', when there is a conflict of interest between the pregnant woman and her unborn child, it is up to the individual conscience to decide upon an abortion or not (WMA, 1970, paras. 2, 3).

That said, even if with time it has been getting easier and easier to obtain an abortion in the light of advances in neonatal care and new abortifacients, the time limit for most types of abortion was lowered in the UK when the Abortion Act 1967 was amended with the Fertilization and Embryology Act 1990. The 1990 Act stipulates that abortion is allowed up to 24 weeks' gestation, except when the mother's life is at risk or the pregnancy is a threat to her mental or physical health or there is a serious risk that the unborn child would be affected by grave abnormality, in which case it is legal up to birth (HFE Act 1990, para. 37 (1)).

While most abortions take place in the first trimester, in practice there is now abortion on demand in Britain – as in many other countries. In the UK there is, however, talk of lowering the 24-week limit further.

WOMEN AND ABORTION

Today the great majority of abortions take place on grounds of the mother's psychological wellbeing, or for what we might call social reasons, rather than her physical health. And the indications for her psychological wellbeing vary from clinically diagnosable psychological conditions to stress through to mere inconvenience caused by the social and familial circumstances in which the pregnant woman finds herself.

Not surprisingly, most abortions are carried out on young unmarried women. According to the UK's Department of Health's abortion statistics relating to England and Wales in the year 2006, the abortion rate was highest at 35 per 1,000 for women aged 19, while overall it was 18.3 per 1,000 in the age-group 15–44.[2] In keeping with these figures, 80 per cent of abortions were carried out for single women. It is also noteworthy that 32 per cent of women undergoing abortions had had one or more previous abortion. As for the timing, 89 per cent of abortions were carried out at or under thirteen weeks' gestation, and 68 per cent under ten weeks' gestation. And it is noteworthy that only 1 per cent of all abortions were undertaken on grounds of foetal abnormality.

The statistics also show that the main medical (non-surgical) method of abortion is the use of the abortifacient drug Mifegyne (Mifepristone, also called RU486). In 2006 some 30 per cent of abortions in England and Wales were early medical abortions. The main surgical methods are vacuum aspiration, which can be used up to fifteen weeks' gestation, and dilation and evacuation (D&E) which is recommended for abortions after the fifteenth week.

In the case of abortions at 22 weeks or later, foeticide is recommended before the procedure takes place. This precaution is noteworthy. It shows that it is now well recognized that the foetus is capable of feeling pain, which raises the question of from what stage of gestation the foetus is capable of feeling pain. Like the ultrasound picture of the unborn child moving, smiling and sucking its thumb, the aforementioned precaution gives pause for thought. Yet, the unborn child counts for what?

If the unborn child really is regarded as a person on a par with its mother, taking its life is a very serious matter. However, both the law and medical practice prioritize the pregnant woman's wellbeing. Is this surprising? The mother is probably a person who is known and loved by a number of other people. She may have parents who love her; she may have a husband and children who love her and need her. How can we not give her preferential treatment, if her life or well-being is threatened by the pregnancy?

The Roman Catholic teaching that abortion is always wrong may seem hard and insensitive in the light of the last-mentioned consider-ations. But its logic is clear. First, it is based on the principle of the sanctity of human (personal) life principle, and the view that the life of a child is a gift. Secondly, it is based on the understanding that good consequences can never justify wrongful means. Moreover, it is argued that, since we cannot tell whether or not the foetus possesses what might be called a personal soul, we must err on the side of caution. Therefore, even if the Magisterium has not dogmatically stated that personal life begins at conception, it teaches that 'the human being must be respected as a person from the very first instant of his exis-tence' (Congregation for the Doctrine of the Faith, 1987, I, para. 1).

Many Evangelical pastors and theologians take an equally firm stand, as witness the strong opposition to abortion in the Bible-belt part of the USA; nor are the pro-life organizations in the UK sup-ported only by Roman Catholics. That said, theologians other than the Catholic ones would tend to take a less absolutist view – though sometimes only marginally so. The renowned twentieth-century American bioethicist Paul Ramsey, a Southern Methodist theolo-gian, defended abortion in order to save the mother's life, though only if both the mother's and the unborn child's lives were at risk (Ramsey, 1968: 81). In other words, he argued that in this situation it is better to save one life than to lose two. In other words, in this sit-uation the physician is acting in a life-promoting way, even if it means sacrificing one life.

The Reformist theologian Karl Barth was only slightly more lenient. Defending abortion in order to save the mother's life, he wrote in his famous work, *Church Dogmatics*, that 'when the choice has to be made between the life or health of the mother and that of the child, the destruction of the child in the mother's womb might be permitted and commanded' (Barth, 1966: 421). His argument was based on compassion for the woman and on the view that she cannot be expected to sacrifice her life for the unborn child. On his reasoning, in this situation, when either the unborn child or the mother has to be sacrificed, the choice to save one is made in the service of life. Hence, the resultant action cannot be regarded as murder (Barth, 1966: 422).

Gilbert Meilaender, a contemporary Evangelical bioethicist, would accept abortion not only to save the life of the mother but also in cases of rape (Meilaender, 1996: 35). Rape raises special questions. Here we have an instance of violation and literal invasion of the woman's body. Indeed, the woman is the victim of a violation of both her bodily and mental integrity, which is why abortion on grounds of rape is often described as a kind of self-defence (Glover, 1990: 131). Even if the child cannot be described as an aggressor, the woman is thought to be defending her bodily integrity. The child is seen as an intruder, even if it is an unwitting intruder. Therefore, how can we ask her to sustain its life? There is a dilemma here, for this very question highlights that the unborn child too is a victim. It is not welcome because it was not conceived in an act of love; it may even be seen as a reminder of the act of violence. Yet some women do learn to love their children so conceived. But, of course, for a woman to offer an unconditional welcome to a child conceived by rape is an act of great generosity. Few women can be expected to have the mental strength or the faith required to accept the life of a child conceived by rape.

Abortion on grounds of rape and abortion to save the mother's life are the hard cases in which even defenders of the principle of the sanctity of life might yield and allow exceptions to the rule. This is because we live in a less than perfect world that does not always leave room for perfect solutions.

Difficult too is the situation in which the unborn child has been found to be affected by a serious medical condition. In this situation, its parents might even feel that they have an obligation to spare it a life of suffering. Glover, a proponent of a quality-of-life ethics, sympathizes with this view (Glover, 1990: 146). The same is true of Singer, though he concedes that 'it must be extraordinarily difficult to cut oneself off from one's child, and prefer it to die, so that another child with better prospects can be born' (Singer, 1995a: 214). Yes, the parents in this sad situation might well have been looking forward to the birth of the child. But instead, in addition to their grief and desire to spare the child a life of suffering, they might fear that they could not cope with a seriously ill or disabled child. They might fear the psychological burden as well as the actual time, effort and financial costs of bringing up such a child. No one should underestimate the difficulty of their situation.

Yet we are faced with the question: if the disabled child is a member of the human family, does it not deserve the same welcome as a healthy child? Put it this way: does the value of a human life reside primarily in health and human abilities? Is it not true that a society which does not welcome disabled members of the human family is one in which many born as well as unborn may be less than safe? Can disabled people feel altogether comfortable in a society which denies life to unborn children on grounds of disabilities which may be similar to their own? These are questions to which we return in Chapter 7.

Having dealt with the difficult cases, it should be noted that these are the exceptions. Few abortions are undertaken to avoid the birth of a disabled child and even fewer on grounds of rape or to save the mother's life. As noted, by far the most common reasons for abortion are psychological or social reasons, relating to the family situation, education or career of the woman. Of course, for the woman to continue her pregnancy might involve great sacrifices even in these situations. She might be a young and unmarried woman who would find it difficult to support and bring up a child on her own. The pregnancy might reduce her chances of finding a husband or partner; it might prevent her from taking up studies; it might interfere with her work or career. Or, if she is a little older and already has a family, she might feel or fear that she could not manage any more children.

One might well sympathize with reasons such as these. But do they justify taking the life of an unborn child? Asking this question is not to imply that women opting for terminations make their choice lightly. Most women having an abortion, be it for social or other reasons, are not ardent pro-choice advocates. Most of them are women who find it hard to cope. If our society were more life-affirming and gave them more support they might not opt for a termination. Our society, which not only sanctions the practice of abortion but also makes it easily available, effectively promotes abortion by treating it as an alternative method of family planning when contraceptives fail. This is arguably both unwise and unkind. An abortion can have adverse consequences for the woman, not just physical ones such as infection, blocked fallopian tubes and sterility, but also psychological ones such as depression (Sutton, 1995: 55–63).

CONCLUSION

The second half of the last century saw a shift in attitudes to and within the medical profession. Secular influences came to dominate much of the debates about medical practices, among them that of abortion. The Hippocratic tradition of medicine lost ground to a new medicine emphasizing quality of life. Abortion was legalized in most countries in the West, and this was not only to save maternal life. Abortion was now allowed under a variety of circumstances.

The old Hippocratic medicine defended by the Roman Catholic Church and also by some bioethicists, doctors and theologians taking a less absolutist view is no longer mainstream. The principle of the sanctity of life and the view that life is always a good has been replaced by a principle of acting with emphasis on quality of life and the view that some lives are not worth living. If this is reflected in discussions about abortion, this is no less true in debates about euthanasia, as will be seen in the next chapter.

CHAPTER 5

EUTHANASIA: QUALITY *VERSUS* SANCTITY OF LIFE

When the prevailing tendency is to value life only to the extent that it brings pleasure and well-being, suffering seems like an unbearable setback, something which one must be freed of at all costs.

John Paul II, 1995, para. 63

INTRODUCTION: EUTHANASIA AND MODERN MEDICINE

Literally speaking, euthanasia means 'easy death' in Greek. Today it is often referred to as mercy killing. Unlike abortion it is a concept that has not received much attention in medical discussion until quite recently, for it is partly the technologization of medicine and the development of modern life-support that has brought the issue of euthanasia to the fore, and partly the new medicine's emphasis on quality of life coupled with an increasing stress on patient autonomy and patients' rights. Coupled with a new sense of patients' rights and an aversion to medical paternalism, demands for euthanasia at the patient's request and physician-assisted suicide may seem reasonable, especially as nobody wants the process of dying prolonged by overly aggressive treatment and technological gadgets. We put our pets down if they are very ill and suffering. We do so because we think it is cruel to do otherwise. How then can we say that it is wrong not to help terminally ill people to die?

The very fact that we can now prolong life in situations when in the past the patient would have died raises the question: when should we stop prolonging life? Once that question is raised, the next question is: when, if ever, should we shorten life? If it is all right to stop making an effort to support life, might it not be most merciful actually to shorten life? Having asked that question we must, after some reflection, also ask: what is the difference between stopping life-support and shortening life? These, then, are the kinds of question that are examined in this chapter.

DEFINITIONS AND LAWS

Euthanasia can be performed by means of a positive intervention such as giving a lethal injection. This would be active euthanasia. It can also be carried out by way of withdrawing or withholding treatment, such as life-support or artificial provision of food and fluids, with the intention to precipitate death. This would be euthanasia by omission, or passive euthanasia.

Given that euthanasia can be carried out both by an active intervention and by an omission, we may define it with reference to the agent's intention to shorten life, as does the British medical doctor and bioethicist John Wyatt. He writes: 'Euthanasia is the intentional killing, by act or omission, of a person whose life is thought not to be worth living' (Wyatt, 1998: 172). This definition is virtually identical to that given by John Paul II in his encyclical *Evangelium Vitae* of 1995, where euthanasia is defined as 'an action or omission which of itself and by intention causes death, with the purpose of eliminating suffering' (John Paul II, 1995, para. 65). Both definitions home in on the intention of the person who brings about the death. This is a widely adopted focus when determining what choices, on the part of doctors, amount to euthanasia and which do not.

However, when people argue in favour of legalized euthanasia, this is usually with a focus on the will of the patient. To make this clear they speak of voluntary euthanasia. Thus what advocates of euthanasia usually have in mind is euthanasia intentionally performed at the patient's own free and informed request. In the Netherlands, the first country to legalize euthanasia and where doctors have long practised it without fear of prosecution, euthanasia is defined as the active and intentional killing of a patient by a doctor at the patient's own request. If the patient did not request help to die, killing him is not called euthanasia. The situation is similar in Belgium, the only other country in the world to have legalized (active voluntary) euthanasia.

The very term voluntary euthanasia implies, of course, that not all euthanasia is undertaken at the patient's request. To be sure, we may distinguish between two different kinds of situation here. We may speak about involuntary euthanasia if the patient is killed against his expressed will or without taking the trouble of finding out what he wants. And we may speak about non-voluntary euthanasia when a patient, who is in no position to express his own wishes, is killed, supposedly in his own best interest or on the assumption that he would want to die.

Involuntary euthanasia is generally considered beyond the moral pale: this is the kind of killing Nazi doctors practised on many disabled people. But even if euthanasia strictly speaking is illegal in the UK, non-voluntary euthanasia by omission has been defended and undertaken in situations in which the patient is thought no longer to have a worthwhile quality of life. The most well-known case – one that has set a trend, though the Law Lords who judged it expressly said it should not – is that of Tony Bland, a young man injured when the Hillsborough football stadium collapsed in April 1989. The seventeen-year-old ended up in a so-called permanent vegetative state (PVS). Patients in this state are unaware of what is going on around them, but they can breathe spontaneously and alternate between a waking and a sleeping state. Tony Bland was kept alive by tube-feeding, but after three years in the PVS state his parents wanted him to be allowed to die. And so, together with their family doctor, they asked the High Court for permission to stop feeding him by artificial means. The case, which received much media attention, went all the way to the House of Lords where the Law Lords decided that it was in Tony Bland's best interest to withdraw the tube-feeding. They decided that it was in Tony Bland's best interest to die, because his life was no longer worth living. So the tube-feeding was withdrawn. It was withdrawn with the express intention that he should die. Tony Bland was deliberately killed by means of euthanasia by omission. For the first time British courts allowed doctors to act to bring about the death of a patient.

But if euthanasia by omission – that is, withdrawal of life-sustaining support with the intention to precipitate death – has effectively been sanctioned in court, active euthanasia remains a crime under UK law.[1] The same remains true of physician-assisted suicide, though maybe not for long. Media coverage suggests that public opinion is swinging in favour of this practice. In the case of physician-assisted suicide, the doctor does not perform euthanasia, he provides the competent patient with the means necessary for the patient to kill himself. The doctor does not kill, but he is an accomplice: he is helping the patient to commit suicide. Like euthanasia, physician-assisted suicide is a criminal offence in most countries. It is, however, legal in Switzerland and the state of Oregon in the United States as well as in Belgium and the Netherlands.

LETTING DIE

If under-treatment is cause of concern, so too is over-treatment. Indeed, fear of over-treatment is one of the reasons why people call for the legalization of euthanasia. As noted by Wyatt, 'the essence of being a good doctor is to know when "enough is enough"' (Wyatt, 1998: 199). Indeed, 'if the burdens of any particular treatment outweigh the benefits, then it should be withdrawn' (Wyatt, 1998: 199). Not to prolong life at all costs is good medical practice, and it is quite different from intentionally hastening death, whether by act or omission.

Wyatt gives the example of a seriously ill cancer patient. Pointing to the burden of chemotherapy, 'with all its unpleasantness, complications, risks, hospital visits', he asks whether it is worth a few extra months of life (Wyatt, 1998: 199). Of course, there is no universally valid 'yes' or 'no' answer to this question. It all depends on the circumstances. For some, but not all, patients, a few extra months of life might be worth the burdens of the treatment required. The decision to provide or withhold treatment has to be made together with the patient and on the basis of an evaluation of the treatment and the value of the extra months of life for the patient. It must not be made on the basis of the value of the patient.

Wyatt makes a distinction between treatment decisions and value-of-life decisions:

> Doctors are qualified to make treatment decisions: to decide which treatment is worthwhile and which is not, but doctors are no better qualified than anybody else to make value-of-life decisions: to decide which life is worthwhile or not. Doctors may determine whether a treatment is futile, but they can never determine whether a life is futile. (Wyatt, 1998: 199)

In other words, a (truly) medical decision to withdraw treatment is based on the belief that the treatment is valueless. It is not based on the belief that the patient is valueless or that his life is valueless.

Wyatt puts the emphasis on the value of the treatment as a means of promoting health and enhancing quality of life. This, rather than an assessment of the value of the patient or of his life, is the deciding factor for doctors who are prepared to let die by withholding or withdrawing treatment, but not prepared to perform euthanasia. On this understanding, a decision to let a patient die is based on an evaluation to the effect that further treatment is futile. The treatment is not withdrawn with the express intention of bringing about death. But death will come. It is the result of the illness. Letting die is to let nature take its course, when further treatment is futile or might lead only to unnecessary pain and prolong the agony for the patient.[2]

That said, there is a debate about what constitutes treatment or not. A distinction is often made between nursing care and treatment, and some bioethicists have argued that the provision of food and fluids should not be considered as treatment but as nursing care. This is because neither food nor fluids can be regarded as medication; others consider artificial provision of food and fluids as treatment because it is invasive. Those in the former camp tend to be slower to sanction the withdrawal of food and fluids, especially the withdrawal of fluids. The Roman Catholic Church's Magisterium, which belongs to this camp, describes the provision of food and fluids as 'an ordinary and proportionate means of preserving life' and says that it is 'obligatory' as long as it accomplishes 'its proper finality, which is the hydration and nourishment of the patient' (Congregation for the Doctrine of the Faith, 2007). In other words, the provision of food and fluids should been seen as ordinary care (or nursing care), unless the patient is incapable of assimilating the food and water or the provision of the same causes too much pain or discomfort. The last-mentioned proviso is important and generally accepted. That is, few disagree with the view that there may come a time when neither food nor fluids should be provided, because the treatment is overly burdensome for the dying patient, or because his body can no longer benefit from it.

PAIN RELIEF AND THE PRINCIPLE OF DOUBLE EFFECT

Not only must euthanasia be distinguished from justified withholding or withdrawal of treatment (including artificial provision of food and fluids), but it must also be distinguished from the provision of sufficient pain relief to terminally ill patients (Wyatt, 1998: 199–200; John Paul II, 1995, para. 65). It is true that drugs used to relieve pain might hasten death – though, very often, they will have the opposite effect because the body gets used to higher and higher doses and also because the patient will be more rested. That said, when such drugs are provided with the intention of relieving pain, death might be foreseen. But it is important to note that death might be foreseen without being intended. Here, as in the case of the removal of a cancerous uterus in order to save the life of a pregnant woman, we must distinguish the intended consequences of the action from any more or less foreseeable or expected consequences not brought about on purpose. Provided the drugs, not the patient's death, are the means of relieving pain, their use can be justified. That is, their use can be justified when alleviation of pain is an overriding concern.

Saying this is not to deny that there could be cases in which it might be hard to determine what the treating doctor's intention really was. But that is a practical difficulty, and not one that invalidates the conceptual distinctions between foresight and intention and between intended and unintended consequences.

REASONS FOR AND AGAINST VOLUNTARY EUTHANASIA AND PHYSICIAN-ASSISTED SUICIDE

As observed by the Australian philosopher and advocate of euthanasia Max Charlesworth, one of the consequences of high-tech medical care is that many people now die in hospital (Charlesworth, 1989: 64–5). And if fear of over-treatment is one reason for calls for legalized euthanasia and/or physician-assisted suicide, so too is the fear of dying not at home but in hospital. Indeed, to the mind of many people the very thought of dying in hospital is as frightening as the thought of overly aggressive medical treatment at the end of life. That is, the thought of dying in an unfamiliar environment surrounded by strangers is as frightening as the thought of a prolonged death.

Despite advances in palliative care and pain relief, many people also fear uncontrollable pain. Fear of pain that cannot be relieved by any means is, then, another reason for demands for legalized euthanasia and/or physician-assisted suicide or guarantees of total sedation in case of unbearable pain.

To meet both the fear of over-treatment and that of pain, the hospice movement, initiated by Dame Cicely Saunders, a devout Christian, has done much to encourage good palliative care with generous pain relief, including self-administration of powerful painkillers such as morphine-derived drugs. The aim of the hospice movement, in the Saunders mould, is to provide care that does not encourage patients to ask for help to shorten their lives. It is to provide care so good and compassionate that no one would want either (voluntary) euthanasia or physician-assisted suicide (Saunders, 1990: 196–205). This aim is based on the belief that often the fears of technological over-treatment and pain, as well as anxiousness about strange and 'unhomely' surroundings, are based more on a fear of the time, place and process of dying than on a fear of death itself. Modern palliative care on this model seeks to help people to live as good a life as possible in friendly surroundings until the end. Quality of life is a prime consideration, but not at the expense of respect for the intrinsic value of every human life. The hospice movement in the Saunders mould promotes quality of life but not by sacrificing the principle of the sanctity of life.

A further reason for requests for the legalization of voluntary euthanasia and/or physician-assisted suicide is the fear of what people describe as a death without dignity. People fear ending up dependent and perhaps not fully *compos mentis*. Many people fear ending up with Alzheimer's and spending their last years in a partially confused state being looked after like a child. They fear what they might call the embarrassment of being helpless and cared for by others. Thus Ronald Dworkin says: 'I want to die proudly when it is no longer possible to live proudly' (Dworkin, 1995: 212).

But is it true that being helpless and in need of care is an indignity? Of course, dementia is a most regrettable state. It means no longer being able to do things one once enjoyed doing; it means losing one's short-term memory. One might forget to eat or be incapable of eating without assistance; one might no longer recognize one's nearest and dearest. From a subjective point of view, this might well seem like an indignity, especially in a society such as ours which puts a premium on autonomy and independence. But this does not mean that persons with dementia have lost their intrinsic human dignity. Thus, as argued by philosophers with sympathies for the old tradition of medicine, people with dementia should be retained within the circle of protection, 'because we remember what they have achieved and we honour their biographical past' (Campbell *et al.*, 2001: 193). Rightly so, for surely those who are ill, dependent and dying remain our fellow humans. As such they never lose their human dignity. Moreover, to accept to be cared for by others is to show trust. It means recognition of the carer as caring and of human community.[3] It is a recognition and acceptance of human sympathy.

Advocates of euthanasia speak, however, of a right to die. They call for respect for patient autonomy. The Australian bioethicist Helga Kuhse, who is a well-known advocate of legalized voluntary euthanasia, holds that:

> Doctors should be permitted to practice voluntary euthanasia because it respects the patient's autonomy and his or her own evaluation of suffering, because it is compatible with sound medical practice (and perhaps required by it), and because there are no good reasons to think that voluntary euthanasia will have bad consequences in practice. (Kuhse, 1996: 257–8)

John Harris agrees:

> To deny people the power of choice over their own destiny is to treat them as incompetent to run their own lives and is thus to make their lives subordinate to our purposes for their lives rather than to treat their lives as their own. (Harris, 1985: 80)

By claiming that patients have a right to be killed, advocates of legalized voluntary euthanasia are effectively saying that medicine in the Christian and Hippocratic tradition is failing the patient who wants to die. This is a frontal attack on the old medicine and the sanctity-of-life principle. It does not go unanswered. Defending the Christian and Hippocratic tradition, John Paul II says: 'Euthanasia must be called a false mercy. True compassion leads to sharing another's pain; it does not kill the patient whose suffering we cannot bear' (John Paul II, 1995, para. 66). Here, then, we are faced with two irreconcilable positions. One upholds the sanctity-of-life principle, the other emphasizes patient autonomy and a right to be relieved of suffering by being helped to die.

Besides the sanctity-of-life argument, opponents of legalized voluntary euthanasia point out that the practice could lead to a lack of trust in doctors. Patients, especially elderly patients, might fear going into hospital lest they should never come out again. It is pointed out that if euthanasia were legalized, elderly patients and those dependent on the care of others could come under pressure to ask for euthanasia from fear of being a burden on relatives or other people.

Furthermore, it is argued that legalized voluntary euthanasia might encourage non-voluntary euthanasia. According to the British bioethicist John Keown, if a doctor is willing to grant a patient's request for voluntary euthanasia on compassionate grounds, he might well think that he ought also to kill other patients with and in the same condition, even if they have expressed no wish to die (Keown, 1992: 88–91; Keown, 2002: 146).

Arguably, the legalization of euthanasia might have even wider ramifications for medicine and society than abortion. If the principle of protecting the weakest members of the human family was first undermined by the legalization of abortion, this was because abortion was not recognized as murder. Calls for legalized voluntary euthanasia are, however, explicit calls for what hitherto has been generally recognized as murder. In short, most advocates of abortion have not regarded the practice as one involving the killing of a person, whereas advocates of euthanasia fully accept that it involves the intentional killing of a person.

ADVANCE DIRECTIVES ABOUT NON-TREATMENT

An advance directive is an advance refusal of certain kinds of treatment made by a mentally competent person. They are made in anticipation of a time when the person is no longer capable of making an informed and competent refusal of treatment. Since April 2007, when the Mental Capacity Act 2005 came into force, such directives are legally binding. That is, such a directive is legally binding provided:

- it is made by a person aged 18 or older; it specifies the treatment to be refused and the circumstances in which the refusal would apply;
- it has not been made under duress and has not been modified verbally or in writing since it was made;
- it has been made in writing and witnessed;
- there is an express statement to the effect that the decision stands even if life is at risk (www.direct.gov.uk).

In an advance directive, then, you may state what treatment you would not want to receive, if in the future you were to lose your mental capacity – but you cannot request any particular kind of treatment, nor can you ask for your life to be ended or force doctors to act against their professional judgement. But, in addition, to legalizing advance directives, the Mental Capacity Act 2005 allows you to appoint an attorney to make health decisions on your behalf if you lose your mental capacity.

The reasoning behind advance directives is based on the recognition of the legal force of treatment refusals made by patients who are *compos mentis*. Indeed, legally speaking it is battery forcefully to treat a mature and mentally sound patient who is refusing treatment. Informed consent must be sought from a patient before he or she is given treatment, especially invasive treatment. In line with this, it is argued that if an adult patient may refuse treatment while *compos mentis*, then he or she should also be allowed to make decisions relating to future non-treatment in case he or she might later lose the ability to make informed choices.

The logic of this argument is obvious, yet many opponents of euthanasia are concerned about advance directives. They fear that such directives might be taken advantage of in order to justify euthanasia by omission, that is, by withholding or withdrawing life-sustaining treatment. Doctors and bioethicists who do not consider the artificial provision of food and fluids as medical treatment voice special concern about the fact that such directives may specify that no food and fluids should be provided by artificial means. Even among doctors who deem the artificial provision of food and fluids as treatment, there are many who consider advance refusals of food and fluids misguided because they fear that such directives might effectively prohibit provision of food and fluids, even in situations when it would be clinically appropriate. In other words, the worry of those concerned about advance directives is that such directives might be used to justify withholding or withdrawing treatment not because it is futile or overly burdensome, but because the patient's life is not considered worth living. In short, there is the fear that advance directives might not only allow doctors to let patients die in peace but also to kill them.

CONCLUSION

We have seen that traditional medicine in the Hippocratic and Christian tradition, which is respectful of the principle of the sanctity of life, is today competing with a new medical ethics. Born in a secular and liberal climate with an overriding concern for quality of life and patient autonomy, this new medicine has little time for the principle of the sanctity of life. Measuring the value of life primarily in terms of its quality, it sees some lives as more valuable than others and some lives as not worth living at all.

Of course, the old tradition is not insensitive to the importance of promoting quality of life. Far from it, those working in the old tradition seek not only to heal but are equally concerned to alleviate pain and promote quality of life when healing is no longer possible. But they will not let concern for the patient's quality of life override the principle of the sanctity of life. They might be prepared to provide pain relief even at the risk of precipitating death, but they will not intentionally perform euthanasia to shorten the patient's life. Therefore, although both traditions speak from a perspective of compassion, their understandings of what compassion requires are very different.

The old tradition is opposed to euthanasia, be it voluntary, non-voluntary or involuntary. The new tradition, on the other hand, is favourably disposed to the legalization of voluntary euthanasia and physician-assisted suicide, at least for patients with terminal or chronic illness. It is so in the name of patient autonomy and the view that quality of life is the prime measure of the value of life.

As will be shown in the next two chapters, the new ethics which puts more emphasis on quality of life than on the intrinsic value of life not only affects attitudes to abortion and euthanasia but also has an impact in other fields of medicine. This is not least in the fields of reproductive medicine and genetics, where some of the new technologies are specifically designed to allow us to select lives on the basis of their quality.

CHAPTER 6

REPRODUCTIVE TECHNOLOGIES AND CLONING

'Now chimes the glass, a note of sweetest strength,
it clouds, it clears, my utmost hope it proves,
for there my longing eyes behold at length
a dapper form, that lives and breathes and moves.
My manikin! What could the world ask more?'
Goethe, *Faust*, Part 2, Act 2, 'Laboratory'
(Goethe, 1969: 101)

INTRODUCTION: PROCREATION OR REPRODUCTION?

In vitro fertilization (IVF) has made thousands of couples happy. It has allowed couples who would otherwise have remained childless to have the child they so much want. Widely welcomed, it has become a routine treatment. Few are questioning its social or moral credentials.

However, the very technique has also allowed us to turn the creation of human embryos into a research project involving their destruction; the very technique has rendered the embryo vulnerable to manipulation. This, then, is a technology that may bring about much good, while also resulting in practices and engendering consequences that are highly controversial. Following in its wake has been research leading to the creation of embryos by asexual means, and by these means even the creation of embryos that are part human and part animal.

If the birth of the first IVF child, Louise Brown, in 1978 broke new ground, even more so did the cloning of the first mammal ten years later. Today we can make a human embryo in a way that does not involve fertilization. Increasingly, human ingenuity has separated what God or nature joined together. With artificial insemination (by husband or donor), which was the first technique of medically assisted conception or artificial reproduction, it became possible to separate sexual intercourse from procreation. With *in vitro* fertilization, meaning 'fertilization in a glass', it became possible not only to separate sexual intercourse from procreation, but also to remove the process of fertilization from the maternal body. The glass dish, not the fallopian tube or womb, became the place where new life begins. With cloning, human-making has gone one step further; it has separated the generation of new life from fertilization. This is a process that is asexual not only in the sense that it involves no mating of man and woman, but also in the sense that it involves no coupling of human gametes.

The term reproduction is therefore apt enough in relation to the new technologies bypassing sexual intercourse. Through the creation of human life by their means, the creation of new life becomes undeniably more like production. If the term procreation suggests the creative involvement of God, the term reproduction might suggest that the child is the product of human-making. And if the idea of the creative involvement of God suggests that the child is a gift, the perception of the child as a product of human-making might suggest that the child-to-be is a chattel. The case is different with techniques such as repair of the fallopian tube allowing couples to have children by normal intercourse, and which are not referred to as techniques of artificial reproduction or artificial fertilization.

Not surprisingly, then, there are those who argue that techniques of so-called artificial reproduction, which bypass 'the union in the flesh', encourage us to see the child-to-be as a product of human design and as such at our disposal to accept or reject. Not surprisingly, there are those who argue that the IVF technology, whereby the embryo is created in the laboratory and which allows us to handle it, encourages us to treat the embryo much as an object. But is it true to say that by-passing sexual intercourse in order to have a child is intrinsically wrong? Is it true that IVF treatment to help a couple conceive a child is wrong as such? Many technologies are, as it were, double-edged.

The prime focus in this chapter is the question of to what extent the new reproductive technologies may affect our attitudes towards nascent human life and children-to-be. That IVF technology has led to research involving the deliberate creation and destruction of human life is clear. Equally, it is clear that IVF treatment has provided much happiness by enabling infertile couples to become parents. In what follows, the last-mentioned fact will not be disputed. Rather, the question is whether or to what extent the new reproductive technologies encourage – or have encouraged – an instrumental attitude towards the embryo and the child-to-be. Is it really true that IVF treatment encourages us to view the child as product of human-making? Does sperm donation encourage us to see the child as a commodity? How do technologies separating gestational and genetic motherhood affect the child and the family?

Since it is impossible to discuss the various technologies without an understanding of the processes involved, we shall begin with a largely descriptive overview of the new reproductive technologies, including cloning.[1] We will then examine some early warnings about the reproductive technologies, warnings to the effect that the new technologies actually do encourage an instrumental attitude to nascent human life. The documents in question are the official responses on the part of the Church of England and the Roman Catholic Bishops of England, Scotland and Wales to the Warnock Committee, as well as the Anglican Oxford theologian Oliver O'Donovan, whose book *Begotten or Made?* published in 1985, was widely discussed at the time and has been influential not least in Evangelical circles. We will also discuss the Roman Catholic Church's Magisterial document, *Donum Vitae*, published in 1987 by the Congregation for the Doctrine of the Faith.[2] This document has had a worldwide impact, in particular on Catholic thinking about the new reproductive technologies.

INFERTILITY AND REPRODUCTIVE TECHNOLOGIES

First used in animal breeding, reproductive technology in the form of artificial insemination was used long before IVF was thought of. Even today it is often used as the first line of treatment in cases of unexplained infertility. As such it usually involves the use of the husband's or the partner's sperm, though to overcome male infertility donor sperm is sometimes used. However, since most couples want a child of their own and not one who is partly the (genetic) child of a stranger, today IVF is often used to overcome not only female but also male infertility.

Who is infertile, then? About one in six couples are infertile in the sense of experiencing difficulty in conceiving. The most common cause of infertility, or subfertility, in men is poor sperm quality. In women most cases of infertility are unexplained, though blocked, or defective, fallopian tubes are a very common cause. Another often mentioned cause is that of polycystic ovaries, which may be precipitated or aggravated by obesity.

A couple is not usually described as infertile unless they have been trying unsuccessfully to have a child for at least two years. Moreover, assisted reproductive technologies (ARTs), that is, procedures which bypass sexual intercourse, are not normally offered unless alternative treatments, such as hormone treatment or tubal surgery to restore normal reproductive functioning, have failed. That said ARTs involving gametal donation might be offered not only in case of infertility but also in order to avoid passing on a genetic condition. What type of ART an infertile couple may be offered depends, of course, on the reason for the treatment.

The main types of ART are: artificial insemination by husband often just referred to as intrauterine insemination (IUI); donor insemination (DI); *in vitro* fertilization (IVF) and related procedures; gamete-intra-fallopian transfer (GIFT). In the UK all procedures involving gametal donation or extra-corporeal conception are regulated by the Human Fertilization and Embryology Authority (HFEA). Procedures such as IUI and GIFT which involve neither extra-corporeal conception nor gametal donation are not regulated under the HFEA. As to surrogacy, it may take two different forms. If the surrogate is artificially inseminated and carries a child for a commissioning couple, the procedure does not fall under the HFEA. But if the procedure involves 'womb leasing' it does, as this means hiring a surrogate to gestate an embryo created by IVF.

IUI

IUI, often the first kind of ART to be used in the case of unexplained infertility, is a simple and pain-free procedure, though sometimes the woman is offered additional fertility drugs (hormones) to stimulate ovulation. The procedure may also be offered if, for example, the man has a low sperm count or if, for some reason, the sperm has difficulty in making its way to the woman's womb. But often IVF is the preferred option in case of low sperm count or poor sperm motility.

DI

DI, with or without hormone treatment, might also be used if there is a male fertility problem. It could also be used if the man has a hereditary disease or has had a vasectomy. In addition, lesbian couples might avail themselves of the procedure. Of course, many people take issue with the last-mentioned practice. Some disapprove simply of gay relationships; others feel that growing up with a lesbian couple is detrimental to the child's psychological development, not least because it deprives the child of a (rearing) father.

As to the question of who can be a donor, in the UK a donor must be aged between 18 and 55, and he is screened for a number of infectious diseases, including HIV, syphilis and hepatitis B. He may also be screened to make sure that he is not a carrier of the gene for cystic fibrosis, the most common genetic disease among people of European origin. But so as not to give the impression of a commercial transaction, the donor is paid no more than £15 plus expenses for each sample provided.

All donor births are registered by the HFEA, and in the case of a married couple the husband is registered as the father on the child's birth certificate, provided he has agreed to the arrangement. However, on reaching 18 the child has the right to obtain information about the identity of the donor. Donor anonymity was removed in the UK in April 2005. This was on the ground that a child has a right to know its genetic origins.[3] Today, then, the HFEA recommends openness with the child from an early age. Yet in reality most couples who have used DI do not tell the child how he or she was conceived.[4]

IVF

Since most couples want a child of their own, IVF using the couple's own egg and sperm is now a more common treatment than DI. That said, older women, aged 40 or more, often have IVF with egg donation. The use of eggs donated by younger women gives them a better chance of becoming pregnant. Occasionally egg or sperm donation might also be used to avoid one parent passing on a genetic disease. Egg donors, like sperm donors, are paid no more than £15 plus expenses. However, many clinics have introduced egg sharing schemes whereby egg donors are offered free or cheaper IVF treatment in return for the donation of some, usually half, of their eggs to another woman. While a woman who has used egg donation is registered as the child's mother on its birth certificate, the IVF child so conceived has the same right to information about the donor as the child conceived by DI.[5] The child produced by egg donation is, however, unique in another respect. It has three biological parents: one genetic father, one genetic mother and one gestational mother.

Today the success rate of IVF is about the same as for natural conception, that is, 20–30 per cent per cycle of treatment. The treatment usually involves hormone stimulation in order to produce several ripe eggs to be fertilized in one treatment cycle. This is to increase the chances of creating a number of embryos to choose from and spare the woman further hormone treatment if her first attempt at IVF fails. That is, healthy embryos – or unfertilized eggs – not used in the first attempt can be stored for future use.[6] If there are healthy leftover embryos that are not stored for future use by the woman, they may be donated to another woman or they may be donated for research.

Egg collection is performed under ultrasound guidance. To avoid discomfort the woman is sedated or totally anaesthetized. After egg collection, the eggs are usually incubated for a short time before sperm – usually obtained by masturbation – are added separately to each egg. Another two or three days later, one or two healthy embryos may be transferred to the uterus by means of a fine tube. If more embryos are transferred there is an increased risk of a multiple pregnancy, that is, a twin or triplet pregnancy, which increases the risk of premature and underweight babies. Sometimes the embryos are tested for a genetic disease such as cystic fibrosis or for a chromosomal condition (such as Down syndrome) before they are implanted in the womb. Most embryos, however, are screened only by microscope inspection.

When there is a problem with the man's sperm, a procedure called intra-cytoplasmic sperm injection (ICSI) may be used. This is a special IVF technique in which a single sperm is injected directly into the centre of the egg. The success rate of this technique is comparable to that of conventional IVF.

While conventional IVF involving hormonal stimulation to make the woman produce several eggs in one cycle remains the most common form of IVF, since the beginning of the century alternative kinds of IVF have been available. Developed primarily to avoid multiple pregnancy, they involve either no hormonal stimulation at all or only minimal such stimulation. These treatments are referred to as natural cycle IVF and mild IVF. Natural cycle IVF, then, involves collecting the egg produced during the woman's natural cycle, whereas mild IVF involves gentle hormone stimulation and egg collection. Not only are these treatments less burdensome for the woman, but they are also less risky. For the main risk associated with IVF is the hormone stimulation, which can have adverse side effects varying from mild discomfort to the life-threatening ovarian hyper-stimulation syndrome. Given that the success rates of the last-mentioned treatments are equal to that of conventional IVF, they have much to commend them.

GIFT and ZIFT

GIFT is in some respects similar to IVF and in other respects more like IUI and DI. It may be used if the woman has at least one func-tioning fallopian tube. Like conventional IVF, it involves hormone stimulation and egg collection. One or two retrieved eggs are then transferred to the fallopian tube together with sperm. Fertilization, therefore, takes place inside the woman's body, which is why the pro-cedure is not regulated under the HFEA, unless gamete (egg or sperm) donation is involved.

ZIFT, short for zygote intra-fallopian transfer, is a similar proce-dure, in which embryos conceived *in vitro* are transferred to the fal-lopian tube. This procedure is regulated under the HFEA.

Surrogacy

The simplest and most common form of surrogacy is that involv-ing artificial insemination, the sperm donor being the male party of the commissioning couple. In this situation the surrogate is both the genetic and the gestational mother of the child. In the case of womb leasing she is only the gestational mother of a child created by IVF using the commissioning couple's gametes. In either case, under UK legislation, a child born as a result of surrogacy is the legal child of the surrogate mother. Thus the surrogate is under no obligation to hand over the child to the commissioning couple. If she gives up the child, the commissioning parents have to adopt it. However, if one or both of them is genetically related to the child they can apply for a simplified adoption procedure, called a parental order.

Commercial surrogacy is illegal in the UK, as is commercial egg and sperm donation. But payment for expenses is allowed and in some cases large sums of money have been changing hands, which effectively turns both the surrogate service and the child into commodities.

CLONING AND HUMAN EMBRYONIC STEM-CELL RESEARCH

Somatic Cell Nuclear Transfer (SCNF)

With the HFE Act 1990 embryo research was allowed by using embryos left over after IVF treatment as well as embryos created specifically for research.[7] This was on the assumption that the embryos created for research were created in the test tube, or Petri dish, with the use of egg and sperm. Cloning to create embryos for research was not yet on the cards. And so, while embryo research could be undertaken to improve fertility treatment or contraception, or to gain a better understanding of the causes of miscarriage or to develop tests to detect genetic and chromosomal abnormalities in pre-implantation embryos (HFE Act 1990, Schedule 2, section 3(1)), there was no mention of cloning in the 1990 Act.

But cloning, that is, somatic cell nuclear transfer (SCNT) to create embryos for research, was soon to become a hot issue. Only six years after the 1990 Act, Dolly the Sheep was cloned. She was the first mammal successfully cloned by SCNT. To be precise, she was created by transferring the nucleus of an udder cell from a six-year-old Finn-Dorset ewe to an enucleated egg, that is, an egg the nucleus of which had been removed (Wilmut, 1997: 810–13). The egg came from another ewe. Born in February 1996 at the Roslin Institute on the outskirts of Edinburgh, Dolly was thus a clone of the six-year-old Finn-Dorset ewe. All her genes, except a few that came from the egg, were identical to the genes of the Finn-Dorset ewe. She was, in all essentials, a genetic copy of the Finn-Dorset ewe.

The technique used is called somatic cell nuclear transfer, because the cell transferred to the enucleated egg in the process is a somatic cell. Soma means body in Greek, so a somatic cell is a body cell, a cell other than sperm or egg cells or their precursors.

Once it had proved possible to clone mammals, scientists were eager to try cloning humans. While this was a controversial issue, it was argued that cloning might lead to novel cures for a variety of diseases. The idea was to clone embryos whose genetic make-up was identical to patients in need of certain kinds of tissue for repair of neural or other damage. The cloned embryos would then be cultured to the stage at which some of their cells, the so-called stem-cells, might be used to create the needed tissue, which would then be transferred to the patient. And as the tissue would be genetically identical to the patient, it was hoped that it would not be rejected as foreign.

But today, so it should be noted, many scientists express the hope that cloning will not be necessary in order to create embryonic-like stem-cell genetically identical to patients. Towards the end of 2007, scientists in Japan and America showed that they had managed to re-wind the biological clock of adult cells, thus turning them into embryonic-like pluri-potent stem-cells.[8]

However, to accommodate embryonic cloning by SCNT for research purposes, which often is called therapeutic cloning, the purposes for which embryo research could be undertaken were extended to allow embryo research to increase knowledge about the development of embryos and about serious diseases, as well as to make such knowledge applicable to treatment for serious diseases. This was under Parliament's Research Purposes Regulations 2001. Cloning to create babies, 'reproductive' cloning, was, however, banned by a separate piece of legislation, namely the Human Reproductive Cloning Act 2001.[9]

Of course, one may well wonder how the transfer of the nucleus of a somatic cell, for example, a skin cell, to an enucleated egg can create an embryo. To explain this, let us look first at what happens when a human embryo is created by fertilization. At normal fertilization a sperm enters an egg and its 23 (gene-carrying) chromosomes link up with the set of 23 chromosomes in the nucleus of the egg. The result is a one-cell human embryo, a zygote, with 23 pairs of chromosomes – that is, 46 chromosomes, 23 from the father and 23 from the mother. When cell division starts each new cell has 23 pairs of chromosomes. Thus human somatic cells (body cells) such as skin cells, muscle cells and neural cells all have 23 pairs of chromosomes in their nuclei. Germ cells (egg and sperm) are exceptions to the general rule, as their nuclei contain only 23 single or non-paired chromosomes.

Now, the entity formed by SCNT, that is, by transferring the nucleus of a human somatic cell to an enucleated egg, has the same number of chromosomes as an ordinary embryo, since the nucleus of a human somatic cell contains 23 pairs of chromosomes. However, its 23 pairs of chromosomes would come, not from a father and a mother, but from a single individual. They would come from the individual whose somatic cell was transferred to the enucleated egg. All its chromosomal genes would come from that individual. With the exception of a few genes that would come with the cytoplasm of the egg used for the procedure, the clone is therefore genetically identical to that individual.

However, while somatic cell nuclear transfer is a sophisticated technique, it is not the transfer itself that is the most amazing part of the cloning procedure. The main trick is that of turning back the biological clock. That is to say, the main trick is to return the adult somatic cell nucleus to an embryonic stage. This is because the new entity is more like the somatic cell used to create it than an embryo. Say the somatic cell used was a skin cell; in a skin cell only skin-cell genes are switched on. By contrast, in a newly formed embryo, the one cell zygote, or the embryo consisting of the first few cells after cell-division has begun, all the genes are switched on. This means that the first cells have the potential to turn into any kind of tissue. But as the embryo grows, its cells begin to differentiate, that is to say, different genes are switched off in different cells. This is how the cells turn into different types of cell.

Thus, to turn the entity created by SCNT into an embryo, non-activated genes must be switched on, which can be done by giving the cell an electric shock or a chemical stimulus. Only when this is done does the new entity start to behave like an embryo. Only then does cell division begin. Only then do we have an embryonic clone.

Therapeutic cloning

In the case of so-called therapeutic cloning, embryos are created by SCNT in order to obtain human embryonic stem cells. These are the cells in the inner cell mass of a five- or six-day-old embryo and the ones from which the 'foetus proper' would develop if the embryo were allowed to continue growing. It is because embryonic stem cells are undifferentiated and so pluri-potential – that is, capable of developing into different kinds of cell – that they are thought to be valuable for research and as a source of repair tissue. Being pluri-potential, they can be used to study the differentiation process of cells and also, so it is hoped, to produce different types of tissue in order one day to treat conditions ranging from Parkinson's disease and Alzheimer's to heart disease and severe burns and spinal cord damage. It is also hoped that cloned embryos created from somatic cells taken from patients with certain diseases will provide new information about the diseases in question.

But if there are scientists who believe that therapeutic cloning provides hope for the future of medical research, this kind of research has many opponents. Many people have moral reservations about this practice, since it involves the destruction of human embryos. Embryo research remains banned in some European countries, among them Austria, Ireland, Italy and Norway. Nor does Germany allow embryo research, though it allows research using imported embryonic stem cells. And while the United States does allow both cloning and embryonic stem cell research, federal funds cannot be used for research on embryonic stem cell lines unless they existed before August 2001.

Not surprisingly the development of embryonic-like human stem cells not produced by cloning but by adding four genes to normal differentiated cells has been warmly welcomed. The new technique, which has been developed by two independent teams, one Japanese and one American, does not involve the creation of an embryo.

The Japanese team of scientists at Kyoto University, under the leadership of Professor Shinya Yamanaka, first tried the technique using mouse cells. Doing so, they rewound the biological clock of adult mouse cells. They created what is termed induced pluri-potent stem cells, or iPS cells for short. This was in 2006. Then in the November 2007 issue of the scientific journal *Cell*, the Japanese team revealed that they had turned back the biological clock of adult human skin cells and so created human embryonic-like pluri-potent stem cells. Only a few days later Professor James Thomson and his Wisconsin University team published a report in the scientific journal *Science* about their creation of human iPS cells.

Both the Japanese and the American teams used viruses to transport four types of gene into human skin cells. And while the scientists don't know how, these genes forced the cells to revert to an earlier pluri-potent stage. Two of the genes used by the two teams were the same, but the other two types were different. Professor Yamanaka used skin cells taken from a 36-year-old woman and from a 69-year-old man, whereas Professor Thomson used immature skin cells taken from a human foetus and from the foreskin of a newborn baby.

Many hail this new technique as the way forward, not least because it is non-controversial, but also because it does not require the use of a human egg. But obstacles remain to be overcome. Most important, as in the case of embryonic stem cells, there is the risk that iPS cell lines could develop into cancer cells. Thus, according to many scientists, for the purpose of medical treatment the use of true adult stem cells remains (at least at present) the safest option.

Adult stem-cell therapy

There is a non-controversial alternative to therapeutic cloning, namely the use of adult stem cells, including umbilical cord-blood stem cells. The use of adult stem cells does not involve the destruction of human embryonic life.

Adult stem-cell treatment has, in fact, been around for a long time. It was pioneered in the 1960s, with transplants of donated bone marrow. Bone marrow transplants, like peripheral blood transplants (blood transfusions), are a type of adult stem-cell treatment. They can be undertaken with donor stem cells (allogenic transplants) or with patients' own cells (autologous transplants). Autologous transplants of bone marrow were initially used to rescue bone marrow from patients due to undergo chemotherapy. Today, autologous peripheral blood stem-cell transplants are used in treatment and in clinical trials involving patients with a variety of diseases, among them breast cancer, myeloma and leukaemia. In fact, autologous stem-cell treatments are now more common than allogenic stem-cell transplantation. However, allogenic bone-marrow transplants are still being used to treat congenital immune deficiencies, bone-marrow failure and sometimes leukaemia (Lennard and Jackson, 2000; Dainiak and Ricks, 2005).

Already in the 1960s it was discovered that bone marrow contains, at least, two kinds of stem cell: haematopoietic stem cells, which normally form the different types of blood cell; and stromal cells which are a mixed cell population, normally generating bone, cartilage and fibrous connective tissue. Today we know that adult stem cells are not only to be found in blood and bone marrow, but can be seen in many kinds of organ and tissue (Rosenthal, 2003). We also know that several kinds of adult stem cell are more versatile than previously thought. That is, we know that some kinds of adult stem cell are almost as pluri-potent as embryonic stem cells. In fact, haematopoietic stem cells may not only follow their normal differentiation paths and generate blood cells, but they may also trans-differentiate into other types of tissue, such as some types of brain cell, including neurons, as well as into skeletal muscle cells, cardiac muscle cells and liver cells. Bone marrow stromal cells too may trans-differentiate into cardiac muscle cells (Kuehnle and Goodell, 2002).

Since there is no question of tissue rejection in the case of autologous adult stem-cell transplants, much hope is placed on autologous treatment using umbilical cord-blood stem cells. Cord-blood banks have therefore sprung up all over the advanced industrialized world. The idea is to store cord blood taken at the birth of a child in case the child might need stem-cell treatment in the future. Of course, autologous stem-cell therapy need not be restricted to stem cells obtained from blood or bone marrow. Today clinical trials are undertaken using patients' own nasal stem cell (olfactory ensheathing cells) to treat spinal cord injuries. With this technique there is hope that people who have suffered paralysing spinal injuries will one day regain the ability to walk.

Other adult stem-cell treatments have already proved highly successful. One such treatment uses donated adult stem cells taken from the eye to restore the sight of people with damaged corneas. There is no problem with foreign tissue rejection, because the foreign stem cells act merely as catalysts triggering the regeneration of the patient's own cells. When their job is done they disappear.[10]

Developments such as these show that real progress is already being made in the area of adult stem-cell therapy. They show that there is no need to go down the avenue of embryo destruction in order to make advances in stem-cell treatment. Likewise, the development of iPS cells gives hope for further stem-cell treatment not involving the creation and destruction of human embryos.

Reproductive cloning

If the cloning technology were perfected, it might be used for 'reproductive' cloning where the clone is transferred to a woman and allowed to be born. Reproductive cloning is, however, widely regarded as immoral. One reason for this relates to the risk of abnormality in the offspring. Most cloning attempts involving mammals have ended in failure. When clones have actually been born, they have more often than not been severely malformed. Cloned animals also age prematurely.

Another reason for objecting to reproductive cloning is that a cloned person would be a copy of another person. This is said to spoil the uniqueness of the person. However, this observation invites the reply that identical twins are not unique either; but cloning is very different from twinning. Unlike clones, identical twins are not copies of another person. Their shared genetic make-up is unique compared with that of other humans.

A third argument against reproductive cloning is that it means making a person to measure. It could be used to create substitutes for dead siblings and copies of megalomaniacs seeking to immortalize their egos. There are, however, those who, like Mary Warnock, argue that cloning could be justified as a form of fertility treatment to avoid genetic illness. If one party of a couple had a serious hereditary disease, the other party could be cloned to give them a child (Warnock, 2002: 102–8).

It may also be noted that a variation of the cloning technique might be used in order to avoid transmission of mitochondrial disease from mother to child.[11] These diseases are hereditary metabolic diseases linked to a few genes found in the cytoplasm surrounding the egg nucleus. The procedure involves the transfer of the cell nucleus of an egg from a woman with the disease to an enucleated egg with sound mitochondrial genes. The reconstructed egg therefore contains the chromosomal genes from the woman with the mitochondrial disease and sound mitochondrial genes from the enucleated egg. While the procedure might be seen as a variation of cloning, it does not result in the creation of an embryo. The reconstructed egg cell must be fertilized *in vitro* to create an embryo. The procedure, which might also be described as a form of egg donation, creates – just like conventional egg donation – a child with three parents: a genetic father and two genetic mothers.

EARLY WARNINGS

In response to the Warnock Committee's discussions and conclusions about the new reproductive technologies and embryo research both the Church of England and the Roman Catholic Bishops in England, Scotland and Wales saw fit to state their views on these issues. Below, these responses are briefly examined in chronological order. We shall then turn to O'Donovan's influential book, *Begotten or Made?* In the UK all these documents were major contributions to the debate on these important subjects.

Last of all we shall discuss the Roman Catholic Church Magisterium's response to the new developments in reproductive medicine. This is a document that has formed the basis for much subsequent literature both for and against medically assisted conception and embryo research.

Catholic Bishops' Joint Committee on Bio-Ethical Issues (1983 and 1985)

The Catholic Bishops' Joint Committee on Bio-Ethical Issues (CBJC) warned already in 1983 that the new reproductive technologies catered to instrumentalist aspirations. In its evidence submitted to the Warnock Committee it said:

A procedure which exploits human knowledge in a way which is seriously inconsistent with true respect for humanity should be excluded from the human community, even if it would contribute to knowledge or some other good end. The principle that human beings are not to be used as mere means to ends of other human beings holds good even when those ends are as worthy and useful as the advance of biological and medical science. (CBJC, 1983: 6)

Thus the Catholic Bishops' Committee strongly objected to embryo research on the ground that, contrary to what is often assumed, the embryo is 'not a potential human being but a human being with potential' (CBJC, 1983: 8).

The Committee also objected to reproductive technologies bypassing sexual intercourse. This was on the ground that the child is treated as a manufacture. In particular, the Committee argued that the child born as a result of IVF comes into being 'as the product of making' and that 'the relationship of product to maker is a relationship of radical inequality, of profound subordination' (CBJC, 1983: 15). This was with the implication that IVF embryo is vulnerable to selection and might be treated as a disposable object if left over after

treatment. According to the Catholic bishops, a truly parental attitude towards the embryo/child is one of unconditional welcome: it
rules out the creation of numerous embryos in the one treatment
cycle and procedures of selection.

The arguments put forward by the Catholic Bishops' Committee
in 1983 were repeated and expanded in the bishops' response to the
Warnock Report published in 1984. As in the earlier document, the
Catholic bishops argued that reproductive technologies bypassing
sexual intercourse turn human generation into a process of production (CBJC, 1985, para. 15). And insisting that 'children have a right
to be born the true child of a married couple, and thus have an unim-
paired sense of identity' (CBJC, 1985, para. 22), they argued that
gamete donation is 'injurious to the rights of the child' (CBJC, 1985,
para. 24).

The Board of Social Responsibility (1984)

Unlike the Catholic bishops' statements, the official Anglican
response by the Board of Social Responsibility (BSR) to the
Warnock Report expressed 'a range of ethical judgements' (BSR,
1984, para. 2.4).[12] Thus the recommendations made by the Anglican
Board of Social Responsibility were expressions of a majority
opinion among the members of the working party. Minority opin-
ions were, however, recorded. In contrast to the Roman Catholic
bishops, the Church of England's working party gave its sanction
to a gradualist approach to prenatal human life. With reference to
the kinds of argument discussed in Chapter 2, the majority on the
working party argued that the early embryo does not deserve the
same respect as the later embryo/foetus.

> The majority of us . . . believe that modern embryology enables
> us to make a judgement of value and believe that (on the view that
> the most probable view should prevail) until the embryo has
> reached the first 14 days of its existence, it is not yet entitled to
> the same respect and protection as an embryo implanted in the
> human womb and in which individuation has begun.
>
> (BSR, 1984, para. 2.7)

Hence, the Anglican working party accepted the Warnock recom-
mendation that embryo research should be allowed up to the end of

the fourteenth day after conception (BSR, 1984, para. 10.6). The majority on the working party also welcomed IVF and artificial insemination. Indeed, they had no problem with these procedures even if they involved gamete donation (BSR, 1984, paras. 5.2, 7.1, 7.2). But 'to promote good family relationships', they did recommend openness with the donor child from the start (BSR, 1984, para. 5.2).

A conservative approach prevailed, however, in the case of embryo donation. This was seen as treating the embryo as a product and commodity (BSR, 1984, para. 8.4). Surrogacy was condemned for the same reason, as well as on the ground that it was an indignity to motherhood, since the surrogate was treated as an incubator (BSR, 1984, para. 9.3). In 1985 the Board of Social Responsibility published a lengthier document, *Personal Origins*, on embryo research and reproductive technology, commenting at length on the 1994 document and explaining the positions taken in greater detail.

While the Church of England's documents expressed less concern about the new reproductive technologies than the documents produced by the Roman Catholic Bishops' Committee, one member of the Anglican Working Party was to speak out with greater reserve.

Oliver O'Donovan's question: begotten or made?

In 1985, Oliver O'Donovan, who had been sitting on the Working Party of the Board of Social Responsibility, published his book entitled *Begotten or Made?* Like the Catholic Bishops, O'Donovan was concerned about the 'producer' attitude to the child. Having been a member of the (conservative) minority group, he expressed the fear that the technological manufacture of embryos might promote an ever more instrumental attitude towards the child-to-be. Comparing the new reproductive technologies with natural intercourse, he said that the child conceived naturally 'is assured by the fact that she is not the primary object of attention in that embrace which gave her being' (O'Donovan, 1984: 17). That is, because the couple are concentrating on one another, the child does not come into being as 'a project pure and simple'; and 'precisely for that reason it cannot be demeaned to the status of artefact' (O'Donovan, 1984: 17).

However, while warning us about the cultural effects of IVF, O'Donovan argued that IVF is not necessarily intrinsically wrong: 'It may even be thought that the cultural influence of the practice is likely to be so bad that IVF should be discouraged for that reason alone ... But ... these cultural questions are different from the question of whether there is something intrinsically disordered about IVF' (O'Donovan, 1984: 79). Indeed, O'Donovan saw nothing intrinsically wrong with IVF, provided the procreational and relational ends of marriage were held together within a loving relationship and the procedure involved neither embryo wastage nor deliberate embryo destruction (O'Donovan, 1984: 17–18). What he feared, however, was that the relationship between the IVF specialist and what he helps to create might encourage an attitude of domination on the part of specialists, parents and, indeed, society as a whole, and thus that the IVF embryo might come to be treated as a disposable object.

> If our habits of thought continue to instruct us that the IVF child is radically equal to the doctors who produced her, then that is good – for the time being. But if we do not live and act in accordance with such conceptions, and if society welcomes more and more institutions and practices which implicitly deny them, then they will soon appear to be mere sentimental, the tatters and shreds which remind us of how we used once to clothe the world with intelligibility. (O'Donovan, 1984: 86)

To be sure, pointing to embryo research, O'Donovan noted that the medical profession and society had, in fact, already taken a big step in the wrong direction. For the IVF embryo used in research is no longer treated as a child-to-be and a fellow human being.

> The practice of producing embryos by IVF with the intention of exploiting their special status for use in research is the clearest possible demonstration that when we start making human beings we necessarily stop loving them; that that which is made rather than begotten becomes something that we have at our disposal, not someone with whom we can engage in brotherly fellowship. (O'Donovan, 1984: 65)

In other words, when we adopt a manufacturer's attitude towards the human embryo, then we alienate ourselves from it.

If O'Donovan had serious reservations about IVF, he was no less concerned about reproductive technologies involving gametal donation. To his mind, even if the sexual bond between the spouses remains intact, because no extra-marital intercourse takes place, the donor is an intruder who drives a wedge between the relational and procreative ends of marriage. And by so doing, he turns the child into an object of barter. For if one undertakes to become a parent 'in order to alienate one's parental relation to the child, one implicitly converts the child to a commodity' (O'Donovan, 1984: 37).

> My argument, then, is that when we narrow our concern for the exclusiveness of marriage to the area of sexual relations, leaving wide-open the field for third-party intervention in procreation, we have taken a fundamental and decisive step towards 'making' our children. We have done it by taking the procreative good of marriage away from its natural root in the exclusive sexual bond of husband and wife. (O'Donovan, 1984: 40)

In short, O'Donovan's book was a strong indictment against an instrumental attitude towards the child or the child-to-be and a clear warning that the new reproductive technologies might lead to an ever more instrumental approach towards nascent human life.

Donum Vitae (1987)

Donum Vitae, published by the Roman Catholic Church's Congregation for the Doctrine of the Faith in 1987, also expressed the fear that ever more technological ways of making children would be accompanied by an increasingly instrumental approach to the embryo and child-to-be: 'Various procedures now make it possible to intervene not only in order to assist but also to dominate the processes of procreation. These techniques can enable man to "take in hand his own destiny", but they also expose him "to the temptation to go beyond the limits of reasonable dominion over nature"' (Congregation for the Doctrine of the Faith, 1987, Introduction, para. 1). Co-signed by Cardinal Ratzinger, the Prefect to the Congregation, and the Congregation's Secretary, Archbishop Alberto Bovone, the document pointed out that there are moral limits beyond which we must not take technology and that the boundaries of these limits are determined by human rights and duties and by respect for human dignity.

On the basis of these observations, coupled with the understanding that 'from the moment of conception, the life of every human being is to be respected' (Congregation for the Doctrine of the Faith, 1987, Introduction, para. 5), it was argued that embryo research and the embryo wastage usually accompanying IVF are beyond the moral pale. The life of the human embryo was said to be 'sacred', because 'from its beginning it involves the creative action of God' (Congregation for the Doctrine of the Faith, 1987, Introduction, para. 5). And against scientists seeking to show that the early embryo is not a human individual, it was argued, with reference to genetic science, that 'from the first instant, the programme is fixed as to what this living being will be . . .' (Congregation for the Doctrine of the Faith, 1987, part I, para. 1). Indeed, it was argued that the human embryo should be treated as a person. For, on the assumption that that the human embryo represents individual human life, it was asked: 'How could a human individual not be a person?' (Congregation for the Doctrine of the Faith, 1987, part I, para. 1).

Yet it was noted that the Magisterium had 'not expressly committed itself' to an affirmation about the personal status of the embryo (Congregation for the Doctrine of the Faith, 1987, part I, para. 1). But Pope John Paul II was later to add that 'what is at stake is so important that, from the standpoint of moral obligation, the mere probability that a human person is involved would suffice to justify an absolutely clear prohibition of any intervention aimed at killing a human embryo' (John Paul II, 1995, para. 60).

Declaring that the child has a right to be conceived, brought into the world and brought up within marriage and that spouses have a right 'to become a father and mother solely through each other', *Donum Vitae* also voiced strong objections to gamete donation (Congregation for the Doctrine of the Faith, 1987, part II, paras. 1–2). Like O'Donovan, the authors of the document described gamete donation as a third-party intrusion and a violation of the marriage bond. And in line with the Catholic Bishops of England, Wales and Scotland, they suggested that donation impinges adversely on the child's sense of identity and could have a destabilizing effect on the family (Congregation for the Doctrine of the Faith, 1987, part II, para. 2).

Indeed, linking their argument to that expressed by Paul VI in his encyclical letter *Humane Vitae* of 1968, the Congregation for the Doctrine of the Faith argued against any form of medically assisted conception which bypasses sexual intercourse. Their argument was based on the understanding of the 'inseparable connection' between 'the unitive significance and the procreative significance' of 'the marriage act' put forward by Paul VI in order to demonstrate the wrong of contraception and show that each single act of (spousal) sexual intercourse should be open to procreation (Paul VI, 1968, para. 12). Not only did Paul VI describe contraception as unnatural in the sense of contrary to the divine order, but he also described it as anti-unitive. That is, he argued that contraception was 'repugnant to the nature of man and woman' and 'strikes at the heart of their relationship', implying that contraception prevents full self-giving (Paul VI, 1968, para. 13). Similarly, the argument presented in *Donum Vitae* suggests that reproductive technologies bypassing sexual intercourse do not involve full spousal self-giving and that marital intercourse alone is symbolically appropriate for the reception of the child as a gift (Congregation for the Doctrine of the Faith, 1987, part II, para. 4: 136). It thus condemns not only technologies involving gamete donation but also IVF and artificial insemination within marriage.

It may, however, be noted that long before *Donum Vitae* was published – but after the publication of *Humane Vitae* – a number of prominent Catholic theologians had made it clear that they took issue with the view that extra-corporeal conception is necessarily wrong. Among them were Richard McCormick (McCormick, 1981: 221–4) and Karl Rahner (Rahner, 1972: 242–51). Those who, like these theologians, argue against the position taken in *Donum Vitae*, say that what matters most is not whether the child is co-created in the warmth of the sexual embrace but whether it is co-created within the warmth of the spousal relationship and is the genetic child of both spouses.

While it is surely not the case that such reproductive technologies are necessarily anti-unitive in the sense of spoiling the spousal relationship, the suggestion that marital intercourse alone is symbolically right for receiving the child as a gift is, however, not to be dismissed as totally meaningless. It implies that by turning conception into a technological process we depersonalize the generation of human life. But, of course, any argument to the effect that the new reproductive technologies are wrong because they are unnatural is weak inasmuch as it suggests that the use of medical technology *qua* artificial is wrong. All medical interventions are unnatural on this line of thinking, but their artificiality clearly does not of itself make them wrong.

CONCLUSION

The warnings issued by the Roman Catholic Church and by theologians such as O'Donovan have surely proved prophetic. This is especially true of the IVF technology which has promoted ever more instrumental treatment of the human embryo. IVF treatment may be welcomed inasmuch as it serves the good of helping many couples to create a family, but it also involves embryo selection and embryo wastage.[13] Moreover, the very technology itself has not only facilitated, but it has been a precondition of, embryo research. This is research that has led to the creation of embryos by the asexual means in cloning, which in turn – as is shown in Chapter 7 – has enabled scientists to create embryos that are part human and part animal.

GENETICS, EUGENICS AND INSTRUMENTALISM

> What nature does blindly, slowly, and ruthlessly, man may do provi-
> dently, quickly and kindly. As it lies within his power, so it becomes his
> duty to work in this direction. The improvement of our stock seems to
> me one of the highest objects that we can reasonably attempt.
>
> Francis Galton, *Eugenics: Its Definition, Scope and Aims*
> (Galton, 1904: 2)

INTRODUCTION: HEALING, SELECTING AND ENHANCING

The recent mapping of the genetic code that makes us human has
opened up a vast array of new possibilities. Thanks to the sequenc-
ing of the human genome, achieved by the multinational government sponsored Human Genome Project (HGP) in 2000, we have
gained information that may revolutionize medicine. The break-
through will lead to new tests for genetically linked diseases as well
as to new therapies. Many of the new tests will serve to improve the
care for patients affected by a variety of conditions, and many of the
new technologies in the field of genetic engineering will help us to
cure diseases that have hitherto been incurable. These developments
are greatly to be welcomed.

However, new knowledge and new technologies also raise new
ethical questions. In the area of genetics the major ethical issues are
those relating to Francis Galton's hopes and aspirations. Testing
with a view to eliminating certain lives is already an established part
of medical practice. Technologies catering to aspirations to improve
the human stock are in the offing.

Healing is one thing. Indeed, it is the primary end of medicine in the
traditional mould, the secondary end being that of alleviating

symptoms, if healing is not possible. Since the second half of the nine-teenth century, we may add to these ends another end of medicine as a life-promoting practice, namely that of prophylaxis, such as sanitation and vaccination but not the elimination of human life. The avoidance of the births of children affected by certain diseases is not among the traditional Christian and Hippocratic ends of medicine. It belongs to the new medicine: that with focus on a quality-of-life ethics as opposed to a sanctity-of-life ethics. Nor are efforts to enhance certain qualities such as mathematical ability, or to promote traits such as blond hair, within the traditional remit of medicine as a healing tradition.

Yet aspirations of the last-mentioned kind are not novel. The hereditary nature of many diseases and many other mental and physical traits has been known since time immemorial. In about 400 BC, Plato put forward a plan for improving the Athenian stock. This was in Book Five of his work, *The Republic*. Here, using Socrates as his mouthpiece, he spelled out a programme for breeding men and women of the best possible kind for the state. Based mainly on selec-tive mating among the Guardian class, this programme also speci-fied rules for the elimination of unwanted children. Plato, then, was an advocate of both positive and negative eugenics, the former being achieved by selective breeding and the latter by avoiding the births of unwanted offspring or, if that failed, infanticide.

It was, however, Galton (1822–1911), a cousin of Charles Darwin (1809–1882), who in more recent times coined the term 'eugenics', which in Greek means 'of good birth'. And it was Galton who called for 'the general intellectual acceptance of eugenics as a hopeful and most important study' (Galton, 1904: 2). It may be added that Galton and Darwin were not just physically related, they were also intellectu-ally related. Darwin's theory of evolution in terms of natural selection and the survival of the fittest sits well with the concept of breeding. Indeed, in his famous work *On the Origin of the Species*, published in 1859, he compared natural selection to man's selective breeding of horses, dogs and pigeons (Darwin, 1996: 18–37, 69). He said that nature works much like a breeder, and yet not by design but on the basis of random variation within species and selection necessitated by circumstances:

> It may metaphorically be said that natural selection is daily and hourly scrutinising, throughout the world, the slightest variations; rejecting those that are bad, preserving and adding up all that are

good; silently and insensibly working, whenever and wherever opportunity offers, at the improvement of each organic being in relation to its organic and inorganic conditions of life. (Darwin, 1996: 70)

An earlier thinker of importance for developments of family planning in the twentieth and the twenty-first centuries – including large-scale prenatal screening programmes – is Thomas Malthus (1766–1834). Putting forward an argument to the effect that populations tend to increase faster than their means of subsistence, he raised fears of overpopulation and discouraged large families. While he was personally opposed to contraception and abortion, his ideas were seminal for the establishment of the Malthusian League. This was a forerunner of the present-day family planning associations and an advocate of means of avoiding unwanted births such as of contraception, sterilization and abortion.

In our day the term 'eugenics' is associated with coercive state programmes. While history points a long finger at the Nazis, such legally founded state programmes, involving the sterilization of mentally disabled people, criminals and people with epilepsy, were in force in the USA, Canada and many parts of Europe in the first few decades of the twentieth century. In Scandinavian countries such programmes remained in force until the end of the 1960s (Broberg & Roll-Hansen, 1996).

Today, because of the association with the Nazi programme, which took the form of both positive eugenics and negative eugenics, any suggestion to the effect that the spectre of eugenics has not been laid tends to be met not just with consternation but with indignation. Nonetheless, eugenic practices and ideas are still with us. They may not come in the form of enforced sterilizations or non-voluntary euthanasia. No, they mainly take the form of non-coercive negative eugenics by way of prenatal diagnosis and selective abortion on grounds of foetal abnormality (Fukuyama, 2002: 84–8; King, 1997: 71–82; Song, 2002: 47–51). Women are not forced to undergo any particular prenatal tests. Reproductive choices involving prenatal diagnosis are voluntary. But there are subtle pressures to undergo such tests. Indeed, the practice of prenatal testing deserves to be called eugenic. Not only is it socially encouraged by ideological pressures to prevent the births of disabled children, but it is also sponsored by health services and regulated by national legislation.

In addition to prenatal testing, medical advances in the area of genetic engineering may encourage eugenic aspirations to improve future generations. But while anyone would hail new ways of curing individuals of genetic diseases, efforts of genetic engineering aimed at promoting traits such as blond hair and mathematical ability raise questions about the rights of future generations not to be made to measure and treated as raw material for us to mould as we like. Even if mental or intellectual characteristics may depend more on nurture than nature, or may be linked to a number of genes making it difficult to modify such characteristics, here the warning of the Christian twentieth-century writer C. S. Lewis is instructive. Writing towards the end of World War II, he warned us not to treat human nature as pure material to be shaped according to human desire and design. In *The Abolition of Man*, he said:

> The final stage is come when Man by eugenics, by prenatal con-
> ditioning . . . has obtained full control over himself. Human
> nature will be the last part of nature to surrender to man. The
> battle will then be won. We shall have 'taken the thread of life out
> of the hand of Clotho' and be henceforth free to make our species
> whatever we wish it to be. The battle will indeed be won. But who,
> precisely, will have won it? (Lewis, 2001: 59)

In Greek mythology Clotho, a goddess of fate, spun the yarn of human life and destiny. Thus by stealing her powers, we would gain the power to make our kind according to our desire and design. 'For the power of Man to make himself what he pleases means', as Lewis says, 'the power of some men to make other men what they please' (Lewis, 2001: 59).[1]

Taking this warning seriously, in this chapter we will discuss the eugenic implications of some of the new technologies and the instrumentalism they may encourage. Looking at the brighter side, we will also consider the new therapeutic possibilities offered by developments in gene engineering.

GENETIC CONDITIONS

Given that all expecting mothers are offered prenatal tests and given the availability of pre-implantation tests in connection with IVF in order to avoid the births of disabled children, it may be helpful to start by explaining what is meant by chromosomal and genetic diseases and how genetic conditions may be inherited.

So what then is a gene? Basically, it is a DNA (deoxyribonucleic acid) sequence. DNA molecules are the double-stranded sequences of four bases that are the building blocks of the 23 pairs of chromosomes found in the nucleus of human body cells. Genes come in pairs (alleles) because chromosomes come in pairs, one of each pair from the mother, the other from the father. The chromosomal make-up of a person is called his or her karyotype. The human male karyotype is 46XY and the human female karyotype is 46XX. The number 46 indicates the total number of chromosomes, while the letters X and Y indicate the sex chromosomes.

The function of genes is to provide the instructions needed by cells for the production of different gene products, usually proteins. Genetic illnesses are caused by malfunctioning genes. Many such malfunctions are hereditary, but some occur *de novo*, that is, they are the result of new genetic mutations. Such mutations may be the result of exposure to toxins or other environmental factors. Genetic disorders such as cystic fibrosis and Huntington's disease are caused by a single malfunctioning type of gene and are inherited from parents. Other genetic conditions may be linked to several types of gene and may be triggered by external conditions such as pollution, eating and drinking habits and other lifestyle factors. This type of condition is called multifactorial or complex. While diseases of this kind have a genetic component, they are not always inherited. Examples of multifactorial conditions are diabetes and heart disease and, no doubt, most of our mental traits.

Since genes come in pairs, provided one copy of the gene is normal the resultant function is usually normal. But in some cases one copy is dominant. The offspring of a person with a dominant copy of gene, such as that for Huntington's disease or adult polycystic kidney disease, has a 50 per cent chance of inheriting the condition. However, in order for a recessive genetic condition like cystic fibrosis to manifest itself, both copies of the gene must be malfunctioning. This means that both parents must pass on a faulty copy of the gene for the child to be affected. When both parents are carriers of a faulty copy of a gene such as this, any offspring of the couple has a 25 per cent chance of being affected.

Some recessive conditions affect some population groups in particular. Cystic fibrosis is the most common recessive condition among people of Western European origin. Sickle-cell disease is most prevalent among people of black African or Arab origin, whereas thalassaemias mainly affect Eastern Mediterranean people and certain Asian groups. It should also be noted that one and the same genetic condition may affect different individuals differently. In addition, some conditions are more penetrating than others, that is, they are more likely than others to manifest themselves distinctly.

A number of conditions are linked to the sex chromosomes, mostly the X chromosome. Since in males the X chromosome is not matched by another X chromosome, but by a smaller Y chromosome, a faulty gene on the X chromosome may not be compensated for on the Y chromosome. This is why X-linked conditions affect only (or almost exclusively) males.

Finally, chromosomal conditions, most of which involve the wrong number of chromosomes, are distinguished from single-gene or multifactorial genetic conditions. Chromosomal conditions may arise at fertilization. This could happen if the egg or sperm has an abnormal number of chromosomes. Such conditions may also arise because of abnormal cell division in the early embryo. The risk of having a child with a chromosomal condition increases with maternal age. The most common condition of this kind is Down syndrome, caused by three copies of chromosome 21, rather than the normal pair. But not all chromosomal conditions involve the wrong number of chromosomes. So-called structural chromosomal conditions are caused by chromosomal breakage and resulting chromosomal rearrangement or some loss of chromosomal material. Some of these conditions may arise *de novo*, others might be inherited.

GENETIC TESTING

Prenatal screening and diagnosis

In the UK all pregnant mothers are offered tests to make sure both mother and unborn child are healthy. Some of these tests are specifically focused on the health of the child. Among them, the Human Genetic Commission (HGC) distinguishes between prenatal screening and prenatal diagnosis. By prenatal screening the HGC understands 'a public health service that offers pregnant women a test to see if the baby is at increased risk of having a particular disorder such as Down syndrome' (HGC, 2006, para. 3.3). Prenatal diagnosis is defined 'as an individual procedure that aims to provide a diagnosis of a particular condition that the baby might have' (HGC, 2006). So the aim of prenatal diagnosis is to determine whether the child actually *is* affected by a certain condition, whereas screening merely indicates a risk. Both tests are undertaken with the aim of promoting 'good births'.

Besides the routine 12-week ultrasound scan to determine dates and later ultrasound scans to look for foetal abnormalities, blood tests with a view to seeing whether the foetus might be affected by a neural defect or a chromosomal condition such as Down syndrome fall under the umbrella term of screening.

When tests such as these indicate that the unborn child might be affected by an adverse condition, further diagnostic tests are offered in order to allow the mother the choice of a termination of pregnancy in case of foetal abnormality. Diagnostic tests may also be offered directly when there is a genetic condition in the family. Many doctors will, however, not offer diagnostic tests unless the woman has indicated that she wants a termination of pregnancy if the unborn child is found to be affected by the condition for which it is tested. This is because diagnostic tests are invasive and involve a certain risk of miscarriage.

The most common diagnostic test is amniocentesis, usually performed between the fourteenth and the twentieth week. Amniotic fluid is obtained by inserting a needle through the mother's abdomen under ultrasound guidance. Since the amniotic fluid contains cells and chemicals of foetal origin, it can be used to detect a variety of genetic conditions as well as non-hereditary conditions such as neural tube defects. But most commonly it is used to detect chromosomal abnormality, the risk of which, as noted above, increases with maternal age and the most common type of which is Down syndrome. As to the risk of miscarrying as a result of this test, it is usually estimated that about 1 in 200 babies are lost in this way.

Chorionic villus sampling, which carries a higher risk of miscarriage, is a less common diagnostic test. According to some estimates, 1–2 in 100 babies are lost after this test (Meire, 2006). Performed between the tenth and twelfth week, it involves a biopsy in order to obtain a small amount of tissue from the pre-placenta (chorion), which contains foetal cells. This test too can be used to detect genetic and chromosomal conditions.

Pre-implantation genetic diagnosis (PGD) and Pre-implantation (chromosomal) screening (PGS)[2]

The IVF embryo is especially vulnerable to selective procedures, as its fate is literally in the hands of its human makers. As explained in Chapter 5, IVF usually involves the creation of several embryos at a time. And since the objective of IVF is to optimize the woman's chance of becoming pregnant and of carrying a healthy child to term, no embryo will be implanted in the womb (uterus) unless it is thought to be sound. Embryos are therefore examined under microscope and sometimes also by more sophisticated means before being implanted. That is, sophisticated tests are available for those who are at special risk of passing on a genetic condition or of having a child with a chromosomal condition.

Thus pre-implantation genetic diagnosis (PGD) is now used to diagnose an increasing number of genetic conditions. The test involves obtaining one or two cells from an embryo about 3 days old, when it may consist of around eight cells. The DNA of the removed cells is amplified and subjected to analysis.

Older mothers, who are at increased risk of having a child with a chromosomal condition, may be offered pre-implantation screening (PGS). This test is used to diagnose chromosomal conditions. Like PGD, it involves the removal of one or two cells from the embryo and testing them for abnormalities, in this case chromosomal abnormalities.

Closer examination of reasons for prenatal and pre-implantation testing

Of course, it is natural for parents to want healthy children. And it is natural for parents to suffer with children affected by serious illness or disability. Thus parents who want to spare their children a life of suffering deserve sympathy. This is not only because a child weakened by illness and needing extra attention and care makes great financial, mental and physical demands on the family. It is because it is terrible to see children suffer.

That said not all foetal conditions for which parents seek, or are offered, terminations involve suffering. Down syndrome children, in particular, are often of a happy disposition and much loved by those around them. More important, who can say whether another person would rather not have been born than be born with a certain disability? Who are you or I to deny life to a child because it suffers from a disability?

Of course, it is true that disability is not good in itself; but a disabled person may nonetheless cherish life. And the disabled person may have much to give. Not only may the person teach us courage, but he or she might teach us to be more humane. As people like this reach out for love and friendship, they may teach us to be more caring. In their very dependence they may teach us to care for others and thus promote a society in which human dignity and value is measured not in terms of economic or social achievement, social status, power or physical beauty and health, but in which the inherent value and dignity of each human being is recognized.

There is, however, an inherently eugenic attitude within our society. Pregnant women are encouraged to have tests to be, as they say, reassured. But the main reason for many tests is to avoid births of disabled children. And so it is pointed out that termination on grounds of foetal abnormality allows couples to embark on new pregnancies, pregnancies that may be unaffected. In addition, it is often emphasized that prenatal diagnosis and selective abortion reduce the mortality rate of infants born with disabilities.

Another reflection of the truth that our society is permeated with a eugenic attitude is the fact that in families with a history of genetic conditions there are often feelings of shame and guilt when a genetic condition is passed on to a child. This suggests a feeling of inferiority among parents with 'bad' genes. Some feelings of guilt may also be explained by the very availability of prenatal screening and diagnosis, which means that the child need not have been born. The very availability of prenatal screening and diagnosis promotes the idea that it is part of responsible parenthood to avoid the birth of a disabled child.[3] In cruder terms, it encourages the idea that we should not welcome unhealthy children – which must send bad signals to those in our society who have been born disabled.

If eugenic aspirations are noticeable in our society, they are even more obvious in societies where boys are favoured over girls and where ultrasound screening coupled with selective abortion is used to choose the sex of the child. In this situation the child is aborted because it is of the wrong sex. But should the child not be welcomed irrespective of its sex? Indeed, should it not be unconditionally welcomed? Moreover, as noted by Francis Fukuyama, although abortion for sex selection is prohibited in China, India and Korea, the practice has already led to severely skewed sex ratios, which is bound to have important social consequences already in the twenty-first century (Fukuyama, 2002: 80–1).

Saviour siblings

The creation of so-called saviour children provides another example of a practice that raises the question of whether a child should not be unconditionally welcomed. A saviour child is an IVF embryo created and tested to serve as a tissue donor for a sick brother or sister. The kind of tissue the parents and doctors would normally have in mind is umbilical cord blood. The test undertaken in order to select a suitable embryo is called (Human Leukocyte Antigen) tissue-typing. It serves to determine whether the embryo's antigens (the molecular markers on its cells that flag them up as the embryo's own and distinguish them from foreign cells) are compatible with those of the sick sibling. What makes this kind of embryo selection controversial is the fact that the embryo found to be a suitable donor is chosen not for its own sake but as a means of healing another child. Even if the saviour sibling later comes to be loved for its own sake, it remains true that it was created to promote the welfare of another.

This puts the child in a situation in which it risks coming under certain pressures (Sutton, 2004). While the initial plan may have been to use umbilical cord blood, it might be tempting to use the child as a bone marrow donor if the umbilical cord blood graft fails. And if that graft also fails, the child might come under pressure to serve as an organ donor. On the worst scenario the child, once it realizes what is happening, might begin to fear for its own safety.[4]

Carrier testing

To turn now to adult testing, carrier testing is undertaken on healthy individuals not with the aim of diagnosing illness but to allow them to find out whether they carry a gene for a disease that could affect their offspring. That is, the aim is to allow people to make 'informed reproductive choices'.

In some societies carrier testing has become the norm before marriage. In Cyprus the state initiated a free carrier testing programme in 1978 in order to reduce the number of births of children with thalassaemia. It may seem surprising, but the programme gained the support of the Church. Since 1981 the Cypriot Orthodox Church has insisted that couples wanting a church wedding must be tested for the condition, which is recessive and so may be inherited by a child when both parents are carriers. Of course, the Church does not stop couples from marrying either in church or outside it. But if both parties are carriers, then they are discouraged from marrying. And if they do marry, they are encouraged by the medical services to undergo prenatal diagnosis with a view to selective abortion of affected offspring (Hoedemaehers *et al.*, 1987: 279–80).

Within the Jewish community in New York there is a similar carrier testing programme aimed at discouraging carriers of Tay-Sachs disease from marrying. This disease is a neurological condition that usually kills the child within the first four years (Bryant and Turnpenny, 2003).

While programmes such as these might be described as eugenic, there is nonetheless a big difference between selective marriages and embryo (or foetal) selection. Selective marriages, if voluntary, may serve as a means of avoiding suffering without sacrificing life. What is controversial, however, is carrier testing linked to policies that limit people's choice of life-partner or policies that put people under pressure to undergo prenatal testing with a view to termination of affected pregnancies.

Predictive testing

Predictive tests are diagnostic in the case of late-onset highly penetrating conditions such as Huntington disease. But in the case of predispositions, such as a predisposition to high blood pressure, they merely indicate a risk.

Aimed at predicting future illness, such tests are mostly offered to adults or older children capable of giving informed consent. That is, the usual aim of such tests is to provide information that may help people to plan for the future. Women with a family history of breast cancer may choose to test themselves in order to know whether they ought to have regular breast-cancer screening. People may also choose to be tested for high blood pressure, diabetes, Crohn's disease or depression, even if tests for these conditions merely indicate a disposition. This is because conditions such as these might be avoided, or their effects might be minimized, by lifestyle choices, such as dieting and exercising.

However, even if predictive tests may allow people to prepare for the future, such tests are not always welcome. To give an example, although a test is available for Huntington disease, few people avail themselves of it. This suggests that many people prefer ignorance to foreknowledge, especially regarding a disease such as this which remains hard to treat.

As for testing children, it is not considered right to burden a young child with information about future illness, unless it is possible to initiate preventive or early treatment. An example of a condition of the last-mentioned kind is phenylketonuria, a recessive genetic disease, for which newborn babies are routinely tested, since the symptoms of the disease may be avoided by putting the child on a special diet.

Exceptionally, a child could also be tested, as could incompetent adults, in order to obtain information needed to promote the health of relatives. This might be justified on the assumption that the incompetent person would have been willing to cooperate, had he or she understood the purpose of the test and provided the test causes no physical harm and little or no mental distress.

CONFIDENTIALITY AND GENETIC TESTING

While it is important to protect the privacy of patients, genetic test results have implications not only for the individual patient but also for other family members. If you are a carrier of the recessive condition cystic fibrosis, then your siblings may also be carriers. And if you test positive for Huntington disease, then one of your parents certainly has the disease and your siblings might have it.

Not surprisingly, then, information about genetic test results can create conflicts of interests within families. A tested patient's concern that the test and its result be kept confidential might clash with the interests of family members who would have welcomed information to help them make informed reproductive or lifestyle choices. Alternatively, relatives given information that they did not ask for might resent it.

Tests might also place medical doctors in difficult situations. The traditional patient-doctor relationship is built on trust and the requirement of confidentiality. But in exceptional circumstances a doctor is obliged to release information in order to protect other people from serious harm. Say the doctor has as a patient a

40-year-old pilot tested positive for Huntington disease but unwilling to give up flying. This patient would pose a grave danger to passengers. Not to warn the employer of the pilot's condition would be irresponsible.

In general, however, it is not correct for a doctor to provide information to employers either about diagnostic or about predictive tests. This is not only because of the requirement of confidentiality but also because tests are often of limited predictive value. Predictive tests for dispositions merely indicate a risk. Indeed, even in the case of a diagnostic test it is often impossible to forecast just how affected the person will be. These considerations are important in discussions about whether employers and insurers should be allowed information about test results.

Not surprisingly there has been much debate about and resistance to the idea of allowing life and health insurers to ask people for genetic test results. Anyone who tested positive for a certain condition would undoubtedly have to pay higher premiums or be refused insurance coverage. Indeed, if insurers were allowed information about test results, discrimination would no doubt ensue. Even the mere knowledge that a person has had a test might put that person at risk of discrimination, since the mere knowledge that the person has taken a test suggests that he or she might be affected by a debilitating condition.

That said, insurers as well as employers sometimes ask and are allowed to know whether there are certain kinds of disease in the family. Arguably there is little difference between asking for such information and asking for predictive test results.

GENE THERAPY

Fifteen years ago people had high hopes about gene therapy and many people thought that it would soon be possible to cure single-gene disorders such as cystic fibrosis, sickle cell disease and thalassaemia. These hopes have, however, not yet been realized, though clinical trials involving transfer of genetic material to patients' bodies for the purpose of treating such conditions are well under way, as are clinical trials involving genetic transfer to cure infectious diseases and heart disease, wounds and, above all, cancer.[5] Indeed, while millions of pounds have been allocated to gene therapy research for treatment of cystic fibrosis, Duchenne muscular dystrophy and other conditions, most clinical gene therapy trials to date have been undertaken for the sake of finding cures for various kinds of cancer. And these have involved a small number of very ill patients for whom there were no other treatment options.

Somatic gene therapy and germ-line gene therapy

An important distinction is made between somatic gene therapy and germ-line gene therapy. The former involves treatment of somatic (body) cells, that is, cells other than reproductive cells. And its effects are restricted to individual patients. The latter affects the reproductive cells, their precursors or the early embryo. The effects of germ-line gene therapy are therefore hereditary.

When people talk about current advances in gene therapy they have in mind somatic gene therapy, which is on a par with conventional treatment inasmuch as it only affects (or is only meant to affect) the individual patient. However, because of concerns about the risks of this relatively novel form of treatment, gene therapy trials in the UK are monitored and regulated by the Medicines and Healthcare Products Regulatory Agency (MHRA), established in 2003, together with the national ethics committee for gene therapy trials, namely the Gene Therapy Advisory Committee (GTAC) set up in 1993 in the wake of recommendations put forward in 1992 by a government sponsored working party, the Clothier Committee, so named after its chairman.[6]

Germ-line gene therapy is prohibited in the UK under the Clinical Trials Regulations 2004. This is on the ground that if anything went wrong, the mistake would be passed on to future generations. Thus, while there is an argument in favour of germ-line gene therapy inasmuch as it might eliminate certain hereditary disorders from whole families and allow them to have unaffected offspring, this kind of therapy is presently deemed too risky. In addition to the risks involved, there are objections to germ-line gene therapy on the lines voiced by C. S. Lewis in *The Abolition of Man*. Individuals affected by germ-line gene therapy would be products of human design with no say in their treatment. And the technology might serve not only to eliminate genetic illness but also to promote or enhance other qualities such as blond hair, athletic build or mathematical ability. Indeed, as suggested by Paul Ramsey some 40 years ago, the technology might even be used 'for man's assumption of control over his own evolution' – which in his view would mean no less than species suicide, that is, the ruin of the human species (Ramsey, 1970: 152).

Genetic enhancement

Interestingly, the World Anti-Doping Agency monitoring athletes is now looking out for so-called gene-doping. That is, it is on the lookout for genetic manipulations aimed at the enhancement of certain physical or even mental characteristics. Why? Because, it is not considered fair play to resort to such technologies in order to improve athletic performance.

Envisaging a future society in which there are two different classes of people, the American bioethicist, Lee Silver, speaks of the GeneRich and Naturals. Belonging to the former class, that of the GeneRich, are people whose genes have been altered to improve their performance in one way or another. Belonging to the class of Naturals are those whose genes have not been altered. The GeneRich, then, are those whose parents could afford to enhance their intelligence and physical performance. The Naturals are the ones whose parents were unable to pay for this luxury (Silver, 2007). In such a world not only would the rich put their children in better schools than the schools in which the poor could afford to put their children, but they would make sure that their children were born with superior potential. You might shudder at the thought. But would this situation be any more unfair than the present one in which some children are placed in better schools than others?

Also, what is the difference between enhancement and healing anyway? We may correct crooked teeth. Is this enhancement or therapy? As noted by Neil Messer, many people consider the distinction between gene therapy and genetic enhancement to be problematic, since the very concepts of health and normality are fluid (Messer, 2003: 91–115). Treatment of crooked teeth might be an example of a borderline case between enhancement and therapy. But while that is true, it is also true that the existence of borderline cases does not mean that there are no clear cases of treatment for disease or no clear cases of non-therapeutic enhancement. While there are good reasons to promote somatic gene therapy, genetic enhancement requires a more cautious approach.

Of course, as noted, we are already enhancing our children by means of education, so why not enhance them by other means? It should, however, be pointed out that genetic enhancement is much more radical than education. Genetic enhancement would mean altering the initial potentials given to our children, whereas education (merely) promotes the potentials they are originally given. In other words, rather than welcoming children unconditionally and helping them to use their natural abilities to their best, genetic enhancement would involve design and a conditional welcome. Children would have to measure up to certain standards, standards imposed, no doubt, partly by cultural fashion and partly by individual parental preferences.

That said, it should also be remembered that we are much more than our genes. We should beware of genetic reductionism. This is particularly true in the case of mental characteristics and personality. To blame all personal shortcomings on our genes or attribute good character solely to our genetic make-up is to deny that we are responsible agents accountable for our actions. It is to deny the existence of a free will. It is to say that our personal development is totally determined by factors beyond our control. But not only is nature coupled with nurture, and not only do we attribute personality to nature and nurture, but we do hold people responsible for their actions and to an extent for their characters. Who and what we are depends not only on our genes. It depends on the womb in which we were gestated, the air we breathe, the food we eat, the upbringing we receive and the people we meet, and something over and above all this, something that we call free will.

Gene therapy procedures

Today we are witnessing rapid and many a welcome development in the field of gene therapy. But before gene therapy can become licensed for routine treatment, there are a number of obstacles to be overcome. A major concern is the risk of side-effects such as development of cancer. Also, the effect of the treatment might be very temporary and so have to be regularly repeated. Moreover, if viral vectors are used for the gene transfer, the patient's body may recognize them as foreign and trigger an adverse immune response. Furthermore, gene delivery has to be precise. Only targeted cells must be affected and they must be affected efficiently. For example, in the case of cystic fibrosis, delivery of healthy genes to cells in the lungs could be difficult because of the presence of mucous. That said, this is a fast developing field.

A common approach is to identify a malfunctioning gene and transfer a functioning copy of that gene to the patient (GTAC, 2007). This can be done either inside or outside the body. It can be done by inserting genes in cells from affected tissue outside the body and then returning the cells to the body. Alternatively, it can be done by delivering the required genes directly *in vivo*, that is, to cells in the body. In either case, the transfer is done with the help of so-called vectors, most commonly viruses. Viruses have the ability to target and enter cells efficiently and they can be rendered harmless by removing viral genes and replacing them with therapeutic genes. Gene transfer may also be done by injecting so-called naked DNA directly into cells. Another possibility involves wrapping the DNA in liposomes (basically fat molecules) to enhance its uptake by cells. Another kind of gene therapy involves gene repair, while yet other techniques may involve switching genes off or the introduction of genes to stimulate the immune system to kill cancer cells.

A related form of treatment, not really to be described as gene therapy, involves the replacement of a missing gene product. Thus when a gene is failing to produce a certain protein, the missing protein itself may be administered. Today there are a number of conditions for which treatment with a missing protein product is improving patients' quality of life.

CONCLUSION

The new gene technologies provide much hope for the future. This is not least in the field of cancer treatment, in which numerous clinical trials are being undertaken worldwide. New treatments are also on the horizon for a number of hereditary conditions. But the idea of improving humankind and creating super-humans with the help of genetic engineering remains a dream – a dream the realization of which would take medical interventions well beyond their present frontiers to the task of helping one generation to design the next.

However, if that is a dream, selection to avoid births of disabled children is part and parcel of modern prenatal care and IVF fertility treatment. Used for diagnostic purposes in order to treat, manage or avoid disease, genetic testing and tissue testing belong within the old tradition of medicine. But this is not so, if they are used for the purpose of eliminating some lives to avoid births of disabled children or to select saviour siblings.

The next two chapters provide further illustrations of novel practices in research and medicine. Some of them serve the traditional aim of medicine, others do not.

CHAPTER 8

ORGAN TRANSPLANTATION, HYBRIDS AND CHIMERAS

An increasing number of moralists – Catholic, Protestant, Jewish and unlabeled men – are manifesting interest, devoting their trained powers of ethical reasoning to questions of medical practice and technology. This same galloping technology gives all mankind reason to ask how much longer we can go on assuming that what can be done has to be done or should be . . .

Paul Ramsey, *The Patient as a Person*, Preface (Ramsey, 1970a: xvi)

INTRODUCTION: WHAT SHOULD BE DONE?

The words above of Paul Ramsey, a renowned bioethicist of the twentieth century, are as applicable today as they were in the 1970s. Indeed today more than ever we must ask ourselves whether all that can be done should be done. Take organ donation. It provides new therapeutic possibilities. At the same time there are dangers, such as abuse of organ donors and a failure to respect the human body and the dead. This is not least because we are confronted with a shortage of organs, a shortage that not only raises questions about different practices of human organ donation but also about the possibility and acceptability of using animal organs and, if so, how far we might go in the direction of using animal tissue in humans. With the arrival of cloning and thus the possibility of transferring a cell nucleus from one cell to another, other altogether new possibilities are opening up, possibilities that in some cases would have been considered science fiction only a few years ago. Indeed, we are now in a position to create organisms that are part human and part animal. But again as always, the question is whether our new technologies are morally acceptable.

In this chapter we shall discuss human-to-human organ donation and also look at the issues relating to the transfer of tissue from one species to another. Thus we shall examine different definitions of death and compare two different legal systems relating to organ donation after death. After that we shall turn to the circumstances under which live donation is legal and may or may not be morally justified. Animal-to-human transplantation is another issue to be discussed before turning in the second part of the chapter to the creation of other kinds of human-animal mixtures. The second part of the chapter, then, deals with human-rabbit and human-cow embryos as well as with mice with human brain cells and other strange creatures whose creation is made possible with modern biotechnology. Here we are clearly faced with the question whether what can be done should be done.

A SHIFT IN ATTITUDE

Needless to say, organ donation raises questions about bodily integrity. This is true in regard to both dead and live donors. Respect for the dead means not treating their bodies as mere raw material. The dead body is more than a potential source of spare parts. As regards living donors, neither on ancient nor on modern understandings is self-harm praised as a virtue. Indeed, the question of bodily integrity is paramount in regard to live organ donors. But what counts as integrity and what counts as self-harm or as unjustifiable self-harm?

Live organ donation is far removed from Hippocratic and traditional Thomist views on what may be done without violating bodily integrity. Not only did the Hippocratic Oath not allow surgery, but according to the Hippocratic principle 'do no harm', any harm done should contribute to the patient's health. But the removal of an organ, say a kidney, from a live donor does not contribute to the donor's health. Similarly, on Aquinas's thinking on bodily integrity, no part of the body may be removed, unless doing so benefits the body as a whole. Therefore if a 'member is healthy and continuing in its natural state, it cannot be cut off to the detriment of the whole' (Aquinas, ST, II, II, q.65.a.1, c.).

Developments in transplant surgery, pioneered in the 1950s, did, however, open up a debate that led Christian as well as Jewish moralists to reconsider their understandings of bodily wholeness and their objections to every kind of bodily mutilation. Once the main medical obstacle to organ donation, that is, organ rejection, had been overcome with the use of drugs to suppress the recipient's immune system, it was difficult to deny the enormous therapeutic potential of organ donation. Kidney transplants – now the most common type of transplant – could clearly transform the lives of people who would otherwise have to spend their lives on and off kidney dialysis machines. Whereas initial organ transplantation surgery had been performed with identical twins as donors and recipients, the new drugs allowed not only transplantation of organs from close relatives to close relatives, but it also became possible to avail of organs from donors unrelated to the recipients. And so a rethink was called for among those opposed to organ donation using live donors, especially as it was soon found that kidneys transplanted from living donors have a better chance of long-term survival than kidneys from dead donors. That said most kidney transplants are from dead donors.

The traditional Catholic principle of totality and integrity, which justified mutilation or injury to a part of the body only for the sake of the person's health, had been formulated with a view to amputation (Jonsen, 2003). Organ transfer from one living person to another was a very different matter, as argued by Jesuit theologian Gerald Kelly, who said it was justifiable as an act of donation and the undertaking of a risk for a proportionate benefit for another (Kelly, 1956). And so the principle of totality came to be modified. A distinction was now made between anatomical wholeness and functional wholeness (Ashley and O'Rourke, 1989: 306). It was argued that the removal of an organ, such as a kidney, could be justified for the sake of saving another, since it is possible for the body to remain functional with one kidney only.

Nevertheless, the idea of permanently injuring a healthy person for the sake of the health of another remained a cause for special caution. One theologian who thought at length about the issue was Ramsey. In his renowned work, *The Patient as a Person*, Ramsey argued that the advantage to the recipient must always outweigh the disadvantage to the donor (Ramsey, 1975: 170–1). This is now taken for granted, although in present-day regulations the strongest emphasis is put on informed consent in the case of the live donors. As for dead donors, the situation is, however, somewhat different as shown below.

DEAD DONORS

Definitions of death

The traditional understanding of death is permanent cardiac stand-still. On this understanding, the patient is considered dead once the heart has permanently stopped beating. However, as a result of modern medical technologies, it is now widely accepted that a person may be dead even if his or her heart is still beating. That is, today a patient may be declared brain dead, even if the heart is beating. Hence, a ventilator may be turned off if the person is no longer thought to be in possession of a functioning brain that would allow the person to continue breathing spontaneously.

You might ask why this is mentioned in the context of organ transplantation. The reason is that many young accident victims who have been declared brain dead end up as organ donors. This is because it is important that organs used for transplantation are both fresh and healthy, and so the question arises of whether the desirability of using donors whose organs are in such a state could lead to the temptation to turn ventilators off too early. The risk of such a temptation might, of course, be minimized by separating the caring team from the transplant team and making sure that the donor is not 'used' until the caring team has turned off the ventilator and the patient has stopped breathing. But these conditions are not – and cannot be – always met. For organs other than kidneys – such as liver, lung and heart – cannot be used unless they are kept perfused with blood until they are removed. Thus the ventilator is not always turned off until the organs for transplantation have been removed, which arguably is a cause for concern. Indeed, some clinicians question whether donors on ventilators really are – or should be considered – dead.[1] To be sure, the very concept of brain death is counter-intuitive. For how can a breathing person whose heart is beating be considered dead? It is hardly surprising that some bioethicists are sceptical about the concept of brain death.[2]

However, even if brain dead patients were no longer to serve as donors, doctors in intensive care units would continue to turn off ventilators in hopeless cases. It should be added that sophisticated medical criteria have been developed for determining brain death. This is so whether doctors use the definition of whole brain death, as they do in the USA and most other countries, or use the British definition of brain-stem death. And it may be noted that, on either understanding, the brain is considered dead only if it is no longer capable of allowing a person to breathe spontaneously. Today, then, not only does the medical profession worldwide accept neurological criteria of death, but the concept of brain death based on the use of neurological criteria has also been accepted by the Churches and by Jewish and Islamic authorities.

That said, some philosophers, among them notably Peter Singer, (Singer, 1995a: 46–54), argue for rather different criteria of brain death than those used to establish total brain death or brain-stem death. They are proposing a cortical definition of death, that is to say, they are suggesting that we should regard a person as dead if he or she is no longer conscious and has suffered permanent loss of all intellectual abilities. This is a controversial view. On this under-standing a spontaneously breathing person in the permanent vege-tative state might be considered dead, which clearly is unreasonable and at odds with any common sense understanding of death.

Opting-in or opting out?

The very term organ donation implies that what is at stake is an act of giving and so a voluntary act. One would therefore assume that organ donation presupposes advance consent on the part of the donor. Today, however, there are different views on what constitutes consent to organ donation on the part of the dead.

Basically there are two different 'consent' systems: the opting-in and the opting-out ones. The opting-in system requires the advance consent of the donor or the consent of his relatives to the removal of organs after his death, whereas the opting-out system requires that those who do not wish to become donors make their refusal to act as donors clear before their death. The last-mentioned system has been devised in response to the shortage of organs and it is based on the idea of presumed consent.

Some opting-in systems are stricter than others. The UK used to have a strict opting-in system in terms of which organs could not be removed from the dead, unless their wishes had been made known before they died. They had to carry a donor card or the like. But in order to make more organs available, this was changed with the Human Tissue Act 2004, applicable in England, Wales and Northern Ireland.[3] Thus relatives can now give consent on behalf of a deceased person if he or she has neither given advance consent nor indicated his or her refusal to donate organs. Alternatively, if the deceased has nominated a person to deal with the use of his body after death, consent can be given by a nominated representative (HTA, 2004, para. 41). In other words, the Human Tissue Act 2004 states that the wishes of the deceased are paramount when – and only when – the person has given advance consent to organ donation. So in this situation, the family cannot intervene and object to donation (HTA, 2004, para. 40). Similar regulations are in force under the Human Tissue (Scotland) Act 2006. In order to meet the demand for organs, we shall probably see further legal changes. Indeed, there are now ongoing discussions about the introduction of an opting-out system in Scotland as well as in England, Wales and Northern Ireland.

There is, however, a clear argument in favour of a strict (or nearly strict) opting-in system inasmuch as it prevents us from treating as a gift what has not been bequeathed as such by the donor (or by relatives of the donor). On the other hand, the disadvantage of an opting-in system, from a public policy point of view, is that it makes fewer organs available for transplantation. That is to say, opting-out systems are based on the assumption that the opting-in system is not in the interest of society at large, given that there is a shortage of organs for transplantation.

Thus, while strict opting-in systems were until recently the norm in the West, today most European countries have an opting-out system. Indeed, all EU-member states except the UK, The Netherlands and Germany have opting-out systems; and Germany is the only country with a strict opting-in system (Nys, 2007: 176). As for the USA, the system varies from state to state. Many states have an opting-out system.

But the question is whether we can really speak of donation and consent in the case of presumed consent. Of course, advocates of the opting-out system might argue that this system puts no less emphasis on the aspect of generosity and giving than an opting-in system. But is that not to take an overly optimistic view of mankind? It is based on the assumption that all of us are willing to donate our organs after death. Clearly that is not the case. Surely the Catholic theologian, David Jones, has a point when saying that: 'The greatest travesty of all is when the state claims the right to use any body that falls into its hands in the name of "presumed consent" ' (Jones, 2001:

62). Arguably, we might speak of stealing rather than donation in this situation.

Not surprisingly, the World Medical Association (WMA) insists that countries with an opting-out system, that is, a presumed consent system 'should make every effort to ensure that these policies do not diminish informed donor choice, including the patient's right to refuse to donate' (WMA, 2006, para. 9). In other words, there is a fear that opting-out systems might take advantage of ignorance by not providing proper information to the public about the right to opt out.

LIVE DONORS

Under what conditions is live donation acceptable?

Obviously donation of a vital organ, such as the heart, is out of the question in the case of live donors. On the other hand, donation of regenerative tissue such as blood and bone marrow or of an organ, such as a kidney which comes in pairs, may be morally licit, provided it does not greatly disadvantage the donor. The risk to the donor should be relatively minor and certainly be outweighed by the benefit to the recipient.

Another requirement, one greatly stressed by most legal systems and in most codes of medical ethics, is informed consent. According to the WMA, living organ donors have a right to information about 'the benefits and risks of transplantation', and, in particular, information about 'the implications of living without the donated organ' (WMA, 2006, para. 17). This means that donors should not only be given an explanation, but they should also be given the opportunity to ask questions and 'should have their questions answered sensitively and intelligibly' (WMA, 2006, para. 20). In addition, 'special efforts should be made to ensure that the choice about donation is free of coercion' (WMA, 2006, para. 20). There should be no more or less subtle pressures in the form of financial incentives. Indeed, in most countries, including the UK, payment for organs is illegal.[4] Not surprisingly, the WMA would like the payment of donors to be prohibited everywhere, since payment might encourage people to take unwarranted risks with their own health (WMA, 2006, para. 23).

As the World Health Organization (WHO) observes, a trade in organs means a commodification of the body; and this is a commodification often accompanied by exploitation (WHO, 2003, para. 11). But, unfortunately, although payment is illegal in almost all countries, there are numerous reports to the effect that 'living donors of transplanted kidneys are remunerated directly or indirectly in many countries' (WHO, 2003, para. 11). Despite the traditional view that organs and tissues should be regarded as gifts, members of the transplant community and policy-makers in several countries have expressed an interest in allowing financial incentives for provision of human body material in the hope of increasing access to transplantation.

Other avenues are also being pursued in order to increase the supply of organs. Until quite recently there was a widely accepted preference for donors genetically related to the recipients, but with the development of drugs to avoid rejection it is increasingly becoming accepted practice also to use donors with an established emotional relationship with the recipients, such as spouses or partners and close friends (cf., HTA, 2006, para. 93). In the UK permission may also be given for certain other arrangements. Thus if the blood group or tissue of a potential donor and recipient are found to be mismatched, the two may be paired with another potential donor and recipient in the same situation (HTA, 2006, paras. 94–96). Such 'paired donations' allow both recipients to receive compatible organs. In some situations more than two donors and recipients may be involved in this kind of swap. To date, however, such 'pooled donations' have been used only for kidney transplants. 'Altruistic donation' is another form of donation whereby a living person may volunteer to donate an organ to an unknown recipient (HTA, 2006, paras. 97–102). Altruistic donors are assessed medically and psychologically. And if they are found suitable their names are placed on a national allocation scheme and matched to a compatible recipient.

Children

It is widely accepted that children and incompetent adults should not normally be used as organ donors. Thus the WMA states that 'individuals who are incapable of making informed decisions, for example minors or mentally incompetent persons, should not be considered as potential living donors except in extraordinary circumstances' (WMA, 2006, para. 23).

Exceptionally, under UK regulations it is, however, possible to remove a solid organ, such as a kidney from a person under 18, if in addition to the child's legal parent's or legal guardian's permission special permission has been granted by the HTA or a court (HTA, 2006, paras. 27–36). To avoid abuse, it is standard practice also to obtain the child's own consent, unless the child is too young to be consulted. Even so it is morally dubious to use children as organ donors, since the removal of a solid organ is medically disadvantageous for the donor. Even donation of bone marrow, which is a regenerative tissue, is controversial, since it is neither entirely risk-free nor painless. Donation of blood, also a regenerative tissue, is another matter, even if it might undeniably cause some minor upset.

As regards a dead child donor, if the child when alive had made a competent decision about donation, the situation is legally the same as in the case of a competent adult. If, on the other hand, the child was too young or if its wishes had not been made known, the parents' or legal guardian's consent must be obtained before an organ can be removed (HTA, 2006, paras. 42–45).

Another contentious issue is the use of foetal donors. As the tissue must be both healthy and fresh, only products of procured abortions can be used for transplant purposes. And while maternal consent might be obtained, the mother's situation may be stressful enough without having to consider whether she should allow her aborted foetus to be used as a tissue donor. A further consideration is the possibility that the very practice of foetal tissue donation might encourage some women to get pregnant and have a termination in order to provide transplant tissue for a relative or a sick sibling or even for herself. Besides, it may be noted that the therapeutic value of foetal tissue is still in dispute, although foetal neural tissue has been used with a degree of short-term success in clinical trials involving patients with Parkinson's disease.

XENOTRANSPLANTATION

One way of meeting the shortage of human organs would be to use animal organs, that is, to start practising xenotransplantation. But initial attempts in the 1960s to transplant kidneys from baboons and chimpanzees to humans failed miserably due to rejection. New hopes were, however, raised in the 1980s with the development of better drugs to suppress the immune system. Thus in 1985 a baboon heart was transplanted to a baby girl – baby Fae – who survived twenty days. The experiment, which took place at Loma Linda Medical School in California, provided encouragement despite the limited success of the operation (Bailey *et al.*, 1985). It may, however, be observed that to date there have been no successful cases of animal-to-human organ donation.

That said, research is being undertaken with pigs in the hope of making it possible to transplant kidneys and hearts from pigs to humans. Pig organs are suitable in size, and pigs are used for human consumption anyway. In addition, they have large litters. Moreover, even if primates are closer to humans, there is a preference for pigs. This is because primates are endangered species and also because it is thought that primates would suffer more than any other animals from being bred as organ donors.

While acute rejection has proved a major problem when transplanting organs from one species to another, some progress has actually been reported (Cooper *et al.*, 2007). Hearts from genetically engineered pigs have been successfully transplanted to baboons which lived for several months without intensive use of immunosuppressant drugs. The achievement was made possible by knocking out a certain pig gene, the gene for alpha-1,3-galactosyltransferate (GT), which is an enzyme found in the blood vessel system of pigs. This made the pig organs more compatible with the baboons, which like humans carry antibodies to GT and, therefore, immediately reject any organ with this enzyme. However, the problem of long-term rejection remained and was manifested by the formation of blood clots in the small blood vessels of the baboons. In other words, there is still some way to go before it is possible to transplant organs from one species to another, and so from animals to humans.

Even if the rejection problem were solved there would remain another major health concern. Indeed, a prime concern in connection with xenotransplantation, and in particular pig-to-human transplantation, is the risk of transmitting infectious diseases from animals to humans. Not only might such diseases be transmitted to individual organ recipients, they might even spread to the wider population. Thus as noted in the *Xenotransplantation Guidance*, published by the Department of Health in 2006, there is a question of public safety. The document reiterates major safety recommendations made by the Council of Europe, the Food and Drug Administration (FDA) in the USA as well as the WHO. Thus it expresses a special concern about certain pig viruses (endogenous retroviruses), which exist harmlessly in pigs, but which could cause diseases in humans and lead to new pandemics.

Animal rights groups have also raised objections to animal-to-human transplantation. UK groups, such as Uncaged and Animal Rights Cambridge, complain about the pain inflicted on animals used in transplant experiments. In particular, they object to the use of apes and monkeys. The American group, People for the Ethical Treatment of Animals (PETA), even describes xenotransplantation as 'Frankenstein science'. Another objection, one often made by the general public, relates to the so-called yuk-factor. Many people say they would not want a pig heart – or any other animal organ. Their feelings are no doubt genuine. But one wonders what they would say if they were in need of a life-saving organ and the only one on offer came from an animal.

That said, a more important concern relates to the integrity of our humanity as a species and to the integrity of the human body as human. The question is whether the recipient of an animal organ might be considered less human than the rest of us? Perhaps it depends on the kind of organ in question? Some organs are more closely associated with our humanity than others. The recipient of a pig heart or a pig kidney would surely remain as human as the rest of us, since these organs perform mechanical functions not specifically related to our humanity. The brain, on the other hand, is of different nature. The human brain is the centre of human self-consciousness and of our intellectual and emotional life. It is essential to our humanity. Thus while a brain transplant is unimaginable, even the transfer of a limited number of brain cells from humans to animals or *vice versa* – which is imaginable – is questionable. Our gonads too are unique and essential to our identity as humans. Indeed, they are inalienable, since the genetic heritage we pass on to our offspring determine their nature and species identity.

HYBRIDS AND CHIMERAS[5]

Today, as noted in Chapter 6, much effort has been invested in embryonic stem-cell research in order to produce various types of tissue with a view to repairing damaged organs and damaged neural tissue. Also discussed was the recent development of so-called induced pluri-potent embryonic-like stem cells, so-called iPS cells. It was noted that the technique used for the production of iPS cells involves neither the creation of embryos nor the use of human eggs and that this renders it non-controversial. That no human eggs are required is also an advantage from a practical point of view, since it is difficult to obtain enough human eggs for cloning to create embryonic stem cells for research. However, the creation of iPS cells is not the only way of compensating for the shortage of human eggs. Another possibility is the use of animal eggs to create human-animal hybrid embryos in order to obtain human embryonic stem cells for research.

The focus in this chapter is on the moral and biological status of human-animal mixtures. A question to be considered is whether such an organism should be described as human if the majority of its chromosomes or cells are human. We must also ask where to draw the line between what should and what should not be done in this field of research.

Apart from human-animal hybrids created for human embryonic stem-cell research, other kinds of animal-human mixtures might be created for pharmaceutical purposes to produce human proteins for medicinal purposes. With our new technologies we can cross the species barrier and create several different kinds of inter-species organisms.

To distinguish between different kinds of mixed species organisms, we use different terms for them. The term hybrid is used for organisms with genes from two or more species within their cells. A chimera is an organism with two or more genetically distinct cell populations. Using this terminology, a human recipient of an animal organ might be called a chimera.

We also speak of different types of hybrids depending on their origin. A true hybrid is an entity created by fertilizing an egg from one species with sperm from another species.[6] A cybrid, on the other hand, is a hybrid organism created by the cloning technique described in Chapter 5. That is, it is created by replacing the nucleus of an egg or cell of one species with the nucleus of a cell from another species. The term 'cybrid' is short for cytoplasmic hybrid. The reason for describing this kind of hybrid as a cytoplasmic hybrid is that it contains a certain amount of cytoplasm from the enucleated egg or cell used to create it. A transgenic organism is yet another type of hybrid created by transplanting a certain amount of DNA (genetic material) from one species to another. Often the transplant is no more than a single gene, but it could even be one or more whole chromosomes.

Our focus here is on the moral and biological status of human-animal mixtures. A question to be considered is whether such an organism should be described as human if the majority of its chromosomes or cells are human. We must also ask where to draw the line between what should and what should not be done in this field of research.

True hybrids

A mule is an example of a true hybrid. It is the product of the mating of a male donkey and a female horse. Every cell of the mule contains genes from both species. True hybrids are rare in nature.

As to the thought of mixing human and animal gametes to create a half-human creature, it is one at which most people shudder. The human revulsion toward sexual involvement with animals, which no doubt is deep-rooted, is clearly marked in the Jewish Bible or the Christian Church's Old Testament (Lev. 18.23). Legally in the UK it is also reflected in the Sexual Offences Act 2003 which prohibits bestiality.

The HFE Act 1990 too bears witness to this revulsion inasmuch as it prohibits the placing of a human embryo in an animal or in an animal cell, as well as the placing of a non-human embryo or non-human sperm in a woman (HFE Act 1990, Section 3(3)). But, nonetheless, the HFE Act 1990 explicitly allows the creation of one kind of true animal-human hybrid. It allows the fertilization of a hamster egg with human sperm – and the development of a two-cell embryo – in order to test male fertility. This is the so-called 'hamster test'. Admittedly, the test is no longer used thanks to the development of ICSI (intracytoplasmic sperm injection). However, the Human Fertilization and Embryology Bill 2007 allows not only the creation of true hybrids by means of the 'hamster test', but it also allows other types of human-animal organisms, including cybrids. It may, however, be noted that many other countries, including Belgium, Canada, France, Germany and the Netherlands, explicitly prohibit the creation of true human-animal hybrids.

Transgenic organisms

The creation of transgenic bacteria and transgenic animals is an established practice for pharmaceutical purposes. Human insulin was the first medication produced by transgenic bacteria. This was achieved by inserting human DNA in E-coli bacteria. Today there are also transgenic animals, such as transgenic sheep, pigs and rabbits that produce human proteins in their milk. Some transgenic sheep and pigs carry human genes for the blood clotting factors VIII and IX. And there are transgenic rabbits which carry genes for interleukin-2, a protein stimulating the proliferation of a certain type of blood-cell, T-Lymphocytes, to fight cancer. Other human proteins produced in the milk of animals are collagen to treat burns, fertility hormones and human haemoglobin, to mention but a few. Even if the animals in question express human proteins in their milk, there is no ambiguity about their animal nature. They remain animals both in appearance and behaviour. What has happened is that tiny bits of DNA (which may have been artificially synthesized rather than obtained from humans) have been spliced into their genome (DNA) for the production of the desired proteins. If the hamster test is controversial, the creation of transgenic bacteria and animals such as the ones just described is surely welcome.

But where do we draw the line or lines in this field of research? There are clearly good reasons to have reservations about certain other types of human-animal mixture. This is not only because some of them might be lethal. To be sure, lethal mixtures create less of a problem than viable mixtures. Take transgenic animals, if too many single foreign genes are transferred to the genome of an organism, it can disrupt its development and even kill the organism. This may well be a blessing. It means that there is probably no need to worry about the possibility of creating transgenic animals with distinctly human features by these means.

But while it might be impossible to transfer a great number of single genes from one species to another, it has proved possible to transfer whole human chromosomes to animals. In this field of research, then, there undoubtedly is a question of where to draw the line.

So what about the creation of an animal-human mixture (a supertransgenic) with one human chromosome? In 2005, UK scientists successfully transplanted the human chromosome-21 into three-day-old mice embryos in order to create a mouse model for Down syndrome (MacKellar, 2007, para. 11.1.2 48–9). The researchers extracted human chromosomes from human cells and sprayed them on to embryonic mouse stem cells. Any stem cells that absorbed human chromosome 21 were then injected into three-day-old mouse embryos, which were successfully implanted into mother mice and born alive with human chromosome-21 in their cells. Moreover, on reaching maturity, they were able to pass on the human chromosome-21 to their young.

The transplanted chromosome, however, did not make the mice in any way human-like. So should we not welcome this kind of research? The ultimate purpose of the research is clearly praiseworthy if undertaken in the hope of finding ways of treating Down syndrome in humans. So are animal-human mixtures created for research by insertion of one or two human chromosomes in the cell-nuclei of animal cells acceptable, provided the organic appearance of the creature is not human-like, and provided the creature shows no human-like behaviour? Perhaps. But how far may we go down this path? Should we choose a 50 per cent fault line? Should we say that provided no more than 50 per cent of the creature's chromosomes are of human origin the research is all right? Are we not on a slippery slope here? From a moral point of view, we are surely moving into deep waters.

There are technical issues too. Should a human-animal organism be said to belong to the animal species if it carries more animal chromosomes than human chromosomes? Where do we draw the line here? Indeed, we are faced with both legal and technical issues. In the UK an embryo falling under the regulations applying to human embryos can be used in research up until the end of the fourteenth day of development or the appearance of the primitive streak. The situation is different for non-human vertebrate embryos. They fall under the Animal (Scientific Procedures) Act 1986, according to which they may be used in research until they reach half the gestation period. Since in mice the gestation period is a mere eighteen days, this means that research involving mouse embryos may be pursued for only nine days. Obviously, this raises questions about the legal time limit for research involving human–mouse mixtures. And it raises questions about what to count as animal and what to count as human. Any line we would draw between animals and humans would be arbitrary. Even a 50 per cent fault line would be arbitrary, not least because there is a problem of determining what weight to give to nuclear DNA compared with mitochondrial DNA.

While issues such as these are being resolved, this field of research remains partly in a legal vacuum. That said, in the UK, the cybrids to which we turn next fall under the regulations guiding human embryo research and so are subject to the 14-day limit.

Cybrids

Already in 1999, the American company Advanced Cell Technologies announced that it had cloned an embryo by inserting the nucleus of an adult human cell into an enucleated cow egg (MacKellar, 2007, para. 12: 52). The embryo was allowed to develop for 12 days. Then in 2003 scientists at Shanghai Second Medical University reported that they had created some 400 human-rabbit embryos and that 100 of them continued to grow for about 4–5 days (MacKellar, 2007, para. 12: 52). These creatures too were created by enucleating an animal egg (in this case a rabbit egg) and then inserting the cell nucleus of a human somatic cell, that is, a body cell, such as a skin cell, as distinct from a reproductive cell. In other words, both types of human-animal embryo were created by somatic cell-nuclear transfer (SCNT), that is, cloning. As a result, some 99 per cent (or so) of their genes (DNA) were derived from the chromosomes in human cell nucleus, while the remaining 1 per cent of DNA was mitochondrial DNA derived from the animal egg.

Every cell in these cybrids was of mixed human and animal origin. The scientists who created them have, so to speak, gone as far down the line as possible. They inserted the full set of human chromosomes in animal eggs. By doing so did they go too far?

From a purely utilitarian point of view, the answer is negative. The creation of these kinds of cybrid may help us to learn more about the process whereby eggs are able to re-programme adult somatic cell-nuclear genes and make them revert to the primitive embryonic stage. It may tell us more about the process of cell-differentiation and about the development of certain diseases. In the future it might even be possible to use human-animal cybrids to create human stem cells for therapeutic use. There is, however, a potential problem here so long as they contain foreign mitochondrial genes. This is because mitochondrial genes of animal origin may prove incompatible with the human body and human genes. In addition, with these kinds of stem cell, as with normal human embryonic stem cells, there is a problem with 'tumorgenicity' – that is, their tendency to turn into cancerous cells.

While the creation of human-animal cybrids may be perfectly acceptable from a utilitarian point of view, the situation is quite different if we hold that human life begins at conception and has a different status than (other) animal life. First, as noted above, most of us have an intuitive revulsion to sexual involvement with animals. And while there is no legal obstacle to the creation of an embryo by placing a human somatic-cell nucleus in an enucleated animal egg, the HFE Act 1990 forbids, as we have seen, the placing of a human embryo in an animal, or in an animal cell, as well as the placing of a non-human embryo or non-human sperm in a woman.

More important, as regards the status of human-animal cybrids, it is noteworthy that scientists wishing to create human-animal embryos by cloning would seem to consider them to be more human than not. Otherwise, why would they regard cow and rabbit eggs as good substitutes for human eggs? This suggests that it is reasonable to describe cloned human-cow and human-rabbit embryonic cybrids as severely compromised human embryos. Legally too these embryos may be assimilated to human embryos, inasmuch as research using these kinds of cybrid is subject to the 14-day limit applicable to human embryo research. Moreover, from a genetic point of view, they are certainly more human than not, since their DNA is nearly 100 per cent human.

If you do count the human embryo as a human being and also hold that personal life begins at conception, you cannot but be concerned about the creation of these compromised human embryos. If this is your understanding, the wilful creation and destruction of compromised human beings must mean treating humans and our species' very humanity as mere raw material to be manipulated and disposed of at will. Moreover, if you believe that humans have a different moral status than animals, you will surely consider it an insult to human dignity to create a compromised human who is part animal and who might therefore be described as a sub-human. Yes, on this understanding, deliberately to create a compromised and lesser human is to add insult to injury. It is insulting and injurious to the creature itself, as well as insulting to human dignity as such. To speak in biblical terms it is to mar the image of God.

If cybrids such as the ones we have been discussing proved capable of pursuing their embryological development, we would also have to ask ourselves a number of probing questions, such as whether we should – or would – treat them as fully human if they developed personal characteristics such as rationality and self-consciousness or any other intellectual or emotional characteristics typical of mature human beings. Would we enter into sexual relationships with them? Would we accept them as equals if they had religious inclinations, political ambitions or commercial aspirations? We would also have to ask ourselves how we should – or would – respond to them if they turned out to be mentally closer to, for example, chimpanzees than humans, but looked as human as the rest of us.

On the understanding that human life begins at conception, the creation of cybrids of the kind discussed cannot be right, since by doing so we would be crossing a Rubicon to a world in which some humans are less than fully human.

Chimeras

Again, to be or not to be human, that is the question. Again, the problem is one of where to draw the line. What does it matter if we place one animal cell or two or even a whole organ in a human body? Does it make the human person any less human? And what does it matter if we place a few human cells in an animal? The answers to these questions depend partly on the type of cell or organ involved.

Animal organs such as kidneys and hearts serve but mechanical functions that in principle might equally well be served by mechanical devices. Apart from the instinctual aversion felt by some, and apart, also, from the medical risks, such transplants should not worry us. The human recipient of a pig heart transplant would indisputably be as human as the rest of us.

But if we think that such organs could be transplanted to humans without making the recipients any less human, we might, as suggested above, feel different about some other types of organ or tissue. Yes, we might feel different about brain tissue or germ-line cells or our sexual organs. The human brain and germ-line cells are intimately associated with our humanity. The human brain is the centre of typically human intellectual abilities. The idea of transplants of animal brain tissue therefore gives pause for thought. The human sexual organs and gametes are if anything even more closely associated with our humanity, since human gametes, human egg and sperm determine the nature and species of our offspring.

Even the introduction of human brain tissue into animals raises serious questions. How would we feel about a creature with the appearance of a mouse or dog, but with distinctly human-like behaviour? While unlikely, the introduction of human brain tissue into an animal brain might create a sub-human creature. Would this not be degrading to humankind? And would it not be both cruel and insulting to the human-like creature trapped in the animal body? Again, to speak in biblical terms, such an experiment would mar the human image of God. And it would be an abuse of our role as stewards appointed to care for other creatures – and our own offspring.

That said, experiments involving the transfer of human brain cells to animals are not only being contemplated, but have already been undertaken (MacKellar, 2007, para. 13.2.2: 58). In 2004, a team headed by Professor Irving Weissman, at Stanford University in the USA, announced that they had injected human progenitor brain cells (neuronal stem cells) into mouse foetuses and thus created mice embryos whose brains were approximately 1 per cent human. The team now wants to inject abnormal human brain stem cells, namely stem cells of the kind causing Parkinson's disease and other neurological conditions, into mouse foetuses in order to study these diseases. *Prima facie*, these experiments might not seem any more controversial than other types of animal research for medical purposes. But, again, where do we stop? Is it all right to create a mouse whose brain tissue is 20 per cent human? Is it all right to create a mouse whose brain tissue is 70 per cent human?

The Stanford team is actually hoping to create mice whose brains are entirely composed of human brain cells. The mouse foetuses would be monitored and, if their brains seemed to develop a human-like architecture, they would be destroyed. If not, they would live on and be used for research. An informal ethics committee has already endorsed the proposal on the ground that human brains cells developing in a mouse cranium are unlikely to create human traits. But, as a precaution, the committee recommended that any (born) mouse showing human-like behaviour should immediately be killed. This is hardly reassuring. The very thought of a self-conscious, more or less rational, creature with more or less human emotions being trapped in the body of a mouse is a grim one. So too is the thought of killing such a creature. Created because it has pleased some scientists to create it, the creature would have cause to consider its human makers cruel and irreverent, lacking in respect both for their own species and for his own compromised humanity. Even if the mice failed to develop human-like behaviour, we would have to say that it was wrong of the ethics committee to give its approval to this kind of experiment, given the fears expressed, since these were fears to the effect that the mice actually might develop human-like behaviour.

The creation of mice with humanlike behaviour sounds, of course, like science fiction. But what is fiction today might turn out to be science tomorrow. This is why we must consider possibilities such as these to avoid being taken by surprise. Some ideas are better rejected before they are realized.

Another such idea – mooted in a report submitted to the House of Lords and House of Commons Joint Committee on the Draft Human Tissue and Embryo Bill, later replaced by the HFE Bill 2007 – is that of transferring human germ-line cells (gonads or reproductive cells) to a certain breed of animals in order for these cells to develop in the animal testes and ovaries and thus allow these animals to conceive and breed humans.[7] The thought of being born not by a woman but by an animal is an abomination, as is recognized in the HFE Act 1990 prohibiting the placing of a human embryo in an animal to be gestated. To deprive some humans of the right to be born by woman would be to deprive them of a fully human heritage and thus of a full sense of human identity.

CONCLUSION

Examining the issue of organ donation involving dead donors, we found both the concept of brain death and the so-called opting-out system controversial. In regard to live donation it was argued that provided the functional integrity, as opposed to bodily integrity, of the donor remains intact, an organ such as a kidney might be donated to save another if the donor has given his full, free and informed consent. The idea of financially remunerated donation was rejected, since payment might lead to exploitation of the poor.

The medical feasibility and ethics of transplanting animal organs into humans was also discussed and this discussion in turn led to a discussion of the status of human-animal hybrids and chimeras. It was concluded that the creation of human-animal hybrids, or so-called cybrids, whose genetic make-up is up to 99 per cent of human origin, effectively means the creation of compromised humans, and that this practice cannot be justified on the assumption that human life begins at conception. It was also argued that the creation of animal chimeras with human brain cells is controversial, because human brain cells are intimately associated with our humanity. As to the creation of a breed of animals with human gonads or reproductive cells, it was noted that this would deprive the human offspring of a sense of being fully human, which would be a grave injustice.

CHAPTER 9

ADULTS AND CHILDREN AS RESEARCH SUBJECTS

So act in that you use humanity, whether in your own person or in the person of any other, always at the same time as an end, never merely as a means.

Immanuel Kant, *Groundwork of the Metaphysic of Morals*
(Kant, 1998: 38)

INTRODUCTION: USE OR ABUSE

The statement by the German Enlightenment philosopher Immanuel Kant, quoted above, may serve as the motto for medical research with human subjects. Used as a research subject the human person does serve as a means to medical and scientific progress, but without such research medical knowledge and expertise would not advance. It is, however, important to remember the intrinsic value and dignity of the human individual and never use him or her as a *mere means*. Taking his rule to say the same as the Golden Rule of the Bible, not to do to others what we would not want them to do to us, Kant would have argued that there are moral limits to medical research on human subjects. Weighing the interests of medical science and the interests of society against the interests of the individual subject of research, we must prioritize the individual lest we allow ourselves to treat the human person as a disposable raw material. The interests of the individual research subject should be second neither to society nor to medical science. Never again should we allow experiments such as those carried out by Nazi doctors on mentally and physically disabled people and people in concentrations camps.

These were experiments that stirred the conscience of the medical profession and so led to the first international code relating to medical research, namely the Nuremberg Code of 1947. Thus after the Second World War the Allies set up courts to try German, Italian and Japanese leaders for crimes against humanity. One of these trials, called the Doctors Trials, ended in 1947 after seven months of testimony. Twenty Nazi doctors and three Nazi medical administrators were charged with murder, torture and other atrocities in the name of science. The Nazi doctors were, however, not alone in having committed crimes of this nature. Japanese doctors had committed similar atrocities during the war. But thanks to a deal struck with the US forces at the end of the war in the Pacific, they were never brought to trial. Nor had the world seen an end to medical atrocities in the name of science and society. While the basic principles of medical research involving human subjects were spelled out in 1947, some nasty experiments later undertaken in the USA were still to come to light.

That said, the Nuremberg Code reflected a new awareness of the duties of the medical profession when testing new procedures and medicines. Although there was no international law to refer to in the Nuremberg trials, the judges argued that the crimes committed were recognized as such by all civilized people and were expressions of natural law. And, needless to say, the Nazis doctors had violated the age-old Hippocratic directive never to inflict harm on patients.

The main person responsible for the writing of the 1947 Nuremberg Code was Dr Andrew Ivy, chosen by the American Medical Association to serve as the prosecution's main medical expert. He spelled out ten basic principles of medical research. These emphasized the duty to obtain the subject's voluntary and informed consent and the subject's right to withdraw his consent at any time. Also stressed was the researcher's obligation to make sure that no death or disabling injury would result and that any risks involved were proportional to, and so outweighed by, the expected benefits of the experiment. In addition, it was declared that no research should be undertaken with human subjects unless prior experiments with animals had been undertaken and unless the results of the research could not be obtained by other means. Furthermore, it was noted that the researcher had a duty to terminate the research if he believed that it might cause harm.

The Nazi experiments had, of course, grossly violated all these principles. Robert Jay Lifton, an American psychiatrist and an expert not only on Nazi genocide but also on the repercussions of the atomic bombs dropped over Japan by the Americans, has described how the sinister medical ideology and practice of the Nazi doctors developed (Lifton, 1987). He tells us how the Nazi eugenics programme involving coercive sterilizations of disabled people led to the killing of 'lives unworthy of living', that is, the killing of disabled adults and children, and eventually to experiments with human 'guinea pigs and genocide' (Lifton, 1986: 22). Over a thousand concentration camp prisoners were infected with malaria and given experimental treatment. Many of them died. Others were infected with jaundice, typhus, cholera, smallpox and diphtheria in studies undertaken to develop vaccines. Battle wounds were simulated and infected. People were starved of oxygen to see how they would react at high altitudes. People were forced to drink salt water. Some were given poisons. Others were sterilized by various methods. The notorious Dr Mengele, who escaped the trials, was especially interested in twins and undertook a number of horrific experiments on twin children. These included the artificial creation of Siamese twins, cross transfusion of blood, exchange of organs from one twin to another and even the deliberate infection of one twin, followed by the killing of both and autopsies.

THE HELSINKI DECLARATION, 1964

In the wake of the Nuremberg Code, the World Medical Association (WMA), founded soon after the war, approved its *Principles for Those in Research and Experimentation*. This was at a general assembly in Rome in 1954. A more detailed declaration, the so-called Helsinki Declaration, was produced in 1964. More strongly worded than the Nuremberg Code, the last-mentioned Declaration – which has undergone several amendments since 1964 – stresses that: 'In medical research on human subjects, considerations relating to the well-being of the human subject should take precedence over the interest of science and society' (WMA, 2004, Article 5). This is a statement that has since been repeated in most national medical research codes worldwide.

Another noteworthy article in the Helsinki Declaration is Article 22, which states that potential research subjects should be told of their right to refuse to participate and to withdraw their consent at any time, without any reprisal. This is another statement that is being echoed in other codes of medical research. Thus it is now widely recognized that abstention from participation in, or withdrawal from, a study should never affect the medical treatment received by the subject. Equally important are Articles 16 and 17, which stress the necessity of weighing risks and benefits and not to undertake research if there are any doubts that the risks to the subjects cannot be managed.

What might be deemed a cause for concern is the fact that the Helsinki Declaration – unlike the Nuremberg Declaration – allows research on persons not capable of giving informed consent. The Declaration does, however, call for special caution in this situation, as it states that informed consent should be obtained from a 'legally authorized representative in accordance with applicable law' and that 'such groups [i.e., people not capable of giving informed consent] should not be included in research unless the research is necessary to promote the health of the population represented and this research cannot instead be performed on legally competent persons' (WMA, 2004, Article 24). In other words, research on people not capable of giving informed consent is said to be permissible only when it is in their own interest or in the interest of people with similar conditions. Thirdly, it is emphasized that 'when a subject deemed legally incompetent, such as a minor child, is able to give assent to decisions about participation in research, the investigator must obtain that assent in addition to the consent of the legally authorized representative' (WMA, 2004, Article 25).

Exceptionally, the Helsinki Declaration also allows research on individuals from whom and in respect of whom it is impossible to obtain consent, including proxy or advance consent. But it is noted that such research should only be undertaken 'if the physical/mental condition that prevents obtaining informed consent is a necessary characteristic of the research population' (WMA, 2004, Article 26). A possible scenario is that of an emergency in which a new treatment might be tried, but in which it is impossible to obtain informed consent from relatives at short notice.

In regard to the testing of new medicines or procedures in the context of medical care, the Helsinki Declaration states that 'the benefits, risk, burdens and effectiveness of a new method should be tested against those of the best current prophylactic, diagnostic and therapeutic methods' (WMA, 2004, Article 29). It is also declared that at the end of a clinical study 'every patient entered into the study should be assured of access to the best proven prophylactic, diagnostic and therapeutic methods identified by the study (WMA, 2004, Article 30). Also noteworthy is the declaration that a refusal to participate in a study 'must never interfere with the patient-physician relationship' (WMA, 2004, Article 31).

UNESCO'S UNIVERSAL DECLARATION ON BIOETHICS AND HUMAN RIGHTS

The United Nations Educational, Scientific and Cultural Organization (UNESCO) is another organization that has spelled out guidelines relating to medical research. It endorses the same basic guidelines as the Helsinki Declaration. In particular, it repeats the statement that 'the welfare of the individual should take priority over that of science and society' (UNESCO, 2005, Article 3.2).

But the organization's focus is not just on the individual subject. The UNESCO document calls for non-discrimination against any groups (UNESCO, 2005, Article 11) and for solidarity and international cooperation (Article 13). It states that: 'Benefits resulting from any scientific research and its applications should be shared with society as a whole and within the international community, in particular with developing countries' (Article 15.1). And it calls for 'special sustainable assistance to, and acknowledgement of, the persons and groups that have taken part in research' (UNESCO, 2005, Article 15, 1.a). This is above all with reference to research undertaken by big multinational pharmaceutical companies in developing countries. In other words, it is a special reminder to those who undertake research on whole population groups in developing countries in order to test new medicines for diseases such as HIV/AIDS or malaria. It is a reminder to treat people in the developing world as our neighbours and not as guinea pigs. If large scale studies are undertaken, the groups involved – both research subjects and controls – should benefit from any findings that might serve their health and wellbeing.

The UNESCO guidelines also urge openness and public dialogue (UNESCO, 2005, Article 15). And, like all more recent guidelines on medical research, they recommend the establishment of ethics committees to scrutinize all research proposals from both a scientific and an ethical point of view (UNESCO, 2005, Article 19).

EU AND UK REGULATIONS

Directive 2001/20/EC of the European Parliament: The EU Clinical Trials Directive

In 2001 the European Parliament adopted its own Directive relating to the implementation of good clinical practice in the conduct of clinical trials involving medical products for human use. This is the EU Clinical Trials Directive, which is binding on all EU member states.

Paying special attention to minors and other incompetent research subjects, and noting the particular need for clinical trials involving children to improve the treatment available to them, the Directive states, in line with the Helsinki Declaration, that such research should only be performed if it could not be undertaken on adults capable of giving informed consent and only if it confers benefit to the subjects involved or others with the same clinical condition (European Parliament, 2001, Article 4.e). Furthermore, it repeats the statement that the wishes of a child capable of informed consent must be respected, thus recognizing the intellectually competent child's right to refuse to take part in a trial (European Parliament, 2001, Article 4.c).

The Directive likewise calls for extra caution in the case of 'incapacitated adults', in particular vulnerable adults such as people with dementia and psychiatric patients. The wishes expressed by a patient while competent must be respected. And if the person is deemed capable of making a decision, his or her wishes must be respected (European Parliament, 2001, Article 5.c). This, then, is a warning to the effect that mentally vulnerable patients should not be abused or taken advantage of.

In addition, there is a special emphasis on the need for independent scientific and ethical scrutiny of all research proposals which should be undertaken by a special ethics committee, that is, 'an independent body in a Member State, consisting of healthcare professionals and non-medical members, whose responsibility it is to protect the rights, safety and wellbeing of human subjects involved in a trial' (European Parliament, 2001, Article 2 (k); Article 3, 2(a)). To be sure the EU Directive refers not only to the obligation of the state to protect the individual, but it also takes note of the accountability of the researcher before society at large. It states that Ethics Committees have an obligation to ensure that there is proper 'provision for indemnity or compensation in the event of injury or death attributable to clinical trials' (European Parliament, 2001, Article 6.h). It is also pointed out that 'all trials must be properly monitored and all results, especially adverse ones, must be recorded in order to ensure the immediate cessation of any clinical trial in which there is an unacceptable level of risk' (European Parliament, 2001, Articles 10; 12).

The Convention on Human Rights and Biomedicine of the Council of Europe

Another inter-European body that has published guidelines for research on human subjects is the Council of Europe. In 2005 it published an additional protocol to the so-called European Bioethics Convention of 1997. The latter laid down broad guidelines on the treatment of human persons in regard 'to the application of biology and medicine' (Council of Europe, 1997, Article 1). The additional protocol, which is closely in line with the European Parliament Directive and the Helsinki Declaration, covers research not only on adults and children but also research on embryos and foetuses *in vivo*.

The Council of Europe additional protocol does, however, not cover research on embryos *in vitro*. This is for the simple reason that the 1997 Convention took a stand against embryo research, allowing it only with the proviso that the embryo received 'adequate protection' (Council of Europe, 1997, Article 18.1). This is noteworthy, inasmuch as the Convention was never signed by the UK, since Article 18.1 of the Convention is in disagreement with UK law. To be precise, Article 18.1 on embryo research states that 'where the law allows embryo research, it shall ensure adequate protection of the embryo', thus excluding embryo research entailing the destruction of the embryo. In addition, the Article states that 'the creation of human embryos for research purposes is prohibited' (Council of Europe, 1997, Article 18.2) – whereas the HFE Act 1990 and subsequent UK legislation, regulating embryo research in the UK, allows not only embryo research, but also the creation of embryos specially for research.

Medicines for Human Use (Clinical Trials) Regulations 2004

While UK regulations are at odds with the Council of Europe's guidelines, it may, however, be noted that the EU's Clinical Trials

Directive of 2001 has been transposed into UK law as the Medicines for Human (Clinical Trials) Regulations 2004. These regulations cover both commercial and non-commercial research involving NHS patients as well as healthy volunteers. A noteworthy effect of these regulations is the requirement that no trial involving medical products may be undertaken, unless it has been approved by an ethics committee and that every such trial must be licensed by the Medicines and Healthcare products Regulatory Agency (MHRA).

The Human Tissue Act 2004

Also to be mentioned here is the Human Tissue Act 2004, which regulates the removal, storage and use of human organs and other tissues in the UK. This legislation was introduced in the wake of shameful events at Bristol Royal Infirmary and the Royal Liverpool Children's Hospital. These events involved the removal and storage of organs from dead children without parental consent. To avoid further offence of this kind, the Act forbids the removal and retention of tissue and organs from the dead for purposes such as education and research, unless proper consent has been obtained either by the deceased before death or by someone nominated by the deceased or someone close to the deceased. As regards living patients, the Act also states that consent must be obtained to the retention and use of their organs and tissue for any purposes beyond diagnosis and treatment. Moreover, all establishments storing human material need to be licensed by the Human Tissue Authority.

SOME BAD EXAMPLES

To bring home how important it is that medical research on human subjects is well regulated, scrutinized and undertaken with the utmost caution and respect for the research subject, a few examples of how not to proceed may be highlighted.

As noted above, the Germans were not alone in undertaking nasty medical experiments. Many other countries must stand accused of undertaking immoral medical research in the first part of the twentieth century (Jonsen, 2003: 125–65). According to a Russian physician, using the pseudonym Vikenty Veressayev, in the first part of the century Russian doctors often deliberately infected institutionalized or chronically ill patients with gonorrhea and syphilis (Jonsen, 2003:

128). These patients were obviously not treated as Kant would have us treat one another, but as mere means in the name of research with no regard at all for their own interests.

The same was true of the research subjects in the American Tuskegee study. Not only were the men involved not told that they were research subjects; they were deliberately deceived about their conditions of health and about what was happening to them. There was no question of voluntary consent. Rather, the nature of the deceit involved constituted a form of pressure or incentive taking advantage of vulnerable people.

The abuse came to light on 26 July 1972, when the *New York Times* carried a report revealing that the United States Public Health Service had for 40 years conducted a syphilis study using 600 black men from Tuskegee, Alabama, as guinea pigs (Jonsen, 2003: 146–8). The research subjects were offered free medical treatment for any disease other than syphilis, as well as a free burial after autopsy. Four hundred of the men suffered from syphilis, but they were neither told about their condition nor offered any treatment. The other 200, who did not suffer from syphilis, were in the control group, the group with whom the syphilis patients were compared. Both research subjects and controls were told that they had bad blood and required regular check-ups. And so when national conscription began in 1941 these men were excluded.

The aim of this research was to study the natural progression of syphilis in untreated patients. Admittedly, when the study began in 1932 the current treatments for syphilis were not very effective. This changed, however, with the discovery of penicillin in the 1950s. Nonetheless, the experiment continued for another 20 years.

An equally unethical study was undertaken at the Willowbrook Hospital in New York for intellectually disabled children (Jonsen, 2003: 153–4; Campbell, Gillet, Jones, 2001: 219). This study was initiated in 1957. Several different kinds of infections were rife at the hospital, one of them viral hepatitis. In order to study the natural course of the disease, researchers set up a special unit in the hospital in which children were deliberately infected with the hepatitis virus.

Contrary to the Helsinki Declaration, but like the Tuskegee study, this research involved neither informed consent, nor any concern for the risks to which the research subjects were exposed. There was no statement to the effect that subjects deemed competent

CHRISTIAN BIOETHICS: A GUIDE FOR THE PERPLEXED

and their legal guardians had the right to refuse consent and to withdraw consent at any time, without the research subjects falling victim
to discrimination in regard to their medical care. It would even
appear that many parents came under pressure to allow their children to partake in the trials, as they were told that their children
would not otherwise be admitted to the hospital (Jonsen, 2003: 153–
4). And while the study did contribute to an improved understanding of hepatitis, it had absolutely nothing to do with the mental
conditions of the children.

These two American studies show the importance of an independent scientific and ethical review of every research proposal, as is
now standard practice. Neither study would have been allowed if
they had been put before a conscientious Ethics Committee.

In the UK, more recent research involving a new drug went dras-
tically wrong with serious repercussions for the research subjects.
Some of them nearly died and one research subject has been maimed
for life. The trial, which took place in 2006, shows that tests on
animals do not always provide a good indication of how humans will
react to a certain drug. It also highlights the need to follow good protocol. Thirdly, it brings to the fore the moral requirement that when
medical experiments or drug trials go wrong the victims should be
compensated.

The trial was special inasmuch as it involved a new type of drug
containing monoclonal antibodies specially designed to trigger an
immune response in humans. The drug, which was intended for
treatment of cancer and rheumatoid arthritis, was tested on animals,
as required by UK regulations. But since it was designed specially for
humans, it was doubtful from the start whether animal tests would
be helpful. As for the protocol, the research subjects should not have
been given the drug so fast one after the other. If the researchers had
allowed more time to elapse after giving it to the first subject, there
would only have been one victim. To add insult to injury, Parexel, the
American group undertaking the trial, sought to avoid talks about
compensation for the suffering and damage to the health of the
affected research subjects. Compounding this problem for the
research subjects was the limited insurance cover of the collapsed
German biotech company TeGenero, which had developed the
fateful drug. While some of the injured research subjects sued
Parexel because they feared that TeGenero's insurance cover would
not be enough to cover their loss of earnings and medical bills, the

worst affected subject was reluctant to take legal action. This was on the ground that legal action for compensation would nullify any claim for compensation from TeGenero.

CONCLUSION

The most fundamental principle of the Helsinki Declaration is that which states that human beings must never be treated as mere means for the sake of medical progress or for the good of science, but that the interest of the individual must always take precedence over the interests of science and society. This principle remains the basic moral rule guiding medical research involving human subjects. While medical research on human subjects is necessary for the progress of medical science, the human being must never be treated as a guinea pig. The human dignity and wellbeing of the subject must always be a prime concern in any trial with humans. Science and technology must serve man, not man science and technology. Thus informed consent is always a requirement in the case of capable adults. In the case of incapacitated adults and minors, the informed consent of legal guardians must be obtained and the subjects' own wishes should always be given serious consideration and, indeed, must be respected if the research subject is deemed capable of giving informed consent. Moreover, incapable adults or minors should not be subjected to medical studies, if these studies can equally well be undertaken on competent adults. This means that presumed consent is never good enough in the context of medical research except in an emergency and the subject is unconscious and the treatment is intended to benefit the research subject.

Finally, all experiments, whether undertaken on competent or incompetent research subjects, must cease immediately if harm results. And those involved in a trial should always be allowed to benefit from any knowledge gained; indeed, if possible, they should be the first to gain.

CHAPTER 10

HOW TO TREAT AND NOT TO TREAT ANIMALS

In answer to James Watson's question: 'What gives a salamander a right?'[1] Francis Fukuyama responds:

> The simplest and most straightforward answer to this question, which applies perhaps not to salamanders, but certainly to creatures with more highly developed nervous systems, is that they can feel pain and suffer. This is an ethical truth to which any pet owner can testify, and much of the moral impulse behind the animal rights movements is understandably driven by the desire to reduce the suffering of animals.
>
> (Fukuyama, 2002: 143)

INTRODUCTION: DO ANIMALS HAVE RIGHTS?

A well-known proponent of animal rights, Peter Singer has told us that the interests of animals should be given equal consideration to that of humans. In his work *Animal Liberation* he writes:

> Many philosophers and other writers have proposed the principle of equal consideration of interests, in some form or other, as a basic moral principle; but not many of them have recognized that this principle applies to members of other species as well as to our own.
>
> (Singer, 1995b: 6–7)

With reference to Jeremy Bentham, the father of the utilitarian rule (according to which we must promote the greatest happiness and the least pain for the greatest number) and who may have been the first to argue for animal rights, Singer says that what matters morally when giving consideration to others, including animals, is whether they can suffer. Quoting Bentham, he says: 'The question is not, Can they reason? Nor, Can they talk? But, Can they suffer?' (Singer, 1995b: 7). Thus noting that Bentham points to the capacity for suffering and enjoyment as the characteristics that give a being the right to equal consideration, Singer writes: 'No matter what the nature of the being, the principle of equality requires that its suffering be counted equally with the like suffering – insofar as rough comparisons can be made – of any other being' (Singer, 1995b: 8). Those who deny this, giving preference to humans, Singer calls specist. And, to Singer's mind, being specist is no better than being racist. But while Singer argues that animals have the same rights as humans to consideration in virtue of their ability to suffer, he also argues – as we have seen when discussing his book *Rethinking Life and Death* – that not all humans have equal rights. For, so he says, some humans are not persons. On his view, babies, for example, are not persons, because they are 'not self-aware, or capable of grasping that they exist over time' (Singer, 1995a: 210). Hence, as we noticed, Singer has suggested that 'a period of twenty-eight days after birth might be allowed before the infant is accepted as having the same right to life as others' (Singer, 1995a: 217). But according to the argument presented here, they obviously have some rights insofar as they are capable of suffering. So what rights are we talking about? Clearly, what is at stake in this context is a right not to be subjected to pain and suffering. In other words, we should inflict no suffering on any sentient creatures.

Surely we agree with Singer that we should seek to avoid inflicting pain on other sentient creatures. Using Christian terminology, we might say that seeking to avoid causing pain is part of our responsibility as God's caretakers. But should we talk of animal rights? Why not, if it is a short-hand for saying that we have no right to inflict pain on animals as we please. Andrew Linzey, an Anglican theologian, argues that animals have 'theos rights'. 'Man and animals form a moral community' (Linzey, 1976: 135), he says. And as God-given life, animals have intrinsic value. Their rights are the other side of the coin compared with our obligations or responsibilities to them before God, as their – and our – giver of life. It is because we humans are superior to animals, spiritually and intellectually, and so 'have a capacity to perceive God's will and to actualize it', that we have these responsibilities (Linzey, 1987: 98). To Linzey's mind, it is possible to 'ground the rights of the creature in the rights of the Creator to have what is created treated with respect' (Linzey, 2002a: 224). Indeed, if animal rights are seen as but counterparts to our obligations as humans aware that animals can suffer, it seems reasonable to speak about animal rights.[2] It may also be granted that animals are part of the giftedness of nature and that they have a value in themselves. Their value does not solely reside in their usefulness to us. Yet few of us would argue that animals have the same rights as humans.

In this chapter we shall discuss the obligations we humans do have to animals, and so by implication their rights. Beginning with a look at the biblical and Christian tradition, we shall examine the obligations implied by the concept of stewardship. We then turn to questions such as whether we ought to be vegetarians and how we should treat farm animals. Hunting is another issue that cannot be ignored, along with the question of animal research, which is the subject on which the chapter closes.

HUMANS AND OTHER CREATURES

In his sermon to the birds St Francis of Assisi speaks of his 'little sisters, the birds,' noting that God preserved their 'seed in the Ark' (Francis of Assisi, 1953: 39). His reference to the birds as his little sisters reflects an attitude of fraternity and respect for animals as co-created inhabitants on Earth, while the reference to the ark of Noah points to our role as stewards, that is, as caretakers responsible before God for how we treat other creatures. On St Francis' understanding, then, animals are seen as our companions, companions towards whom we have a special responsibility before our Creator. Yet they are not our equals. They have no responsibilities towards or for us.

St Francis is often held up as an example of how we should relate to animals. Thus the Catechism of the Catholic Church tells us to 'recall the gentleness with which saints like St Francis of Assisi and St Philip Neri treated animals' (*Catechism*, para. 2416). However, Singer describes St Francis as the exception to the rule within Christianity. Is this right? Singer says that Catholicism in particular, 'discourages concern for the welfare of non-human beings' (Singer, 1995b: 197). Surely, the very reminder just quoted should prove him wrong. But let us look a bit more closely at the biblical and Christian views on our relationship to animals.

On the Old Testament understanding (common to Jews, Christians and Muslims), we humans have a special covenant-relationship with

God, which involves a caretaker responsibility for the rest of creation, including above all other sentient creatures. In the Old Testament animals are brought into the saving presence of God through their relationship with mankind. In Genesis 9, which tells us about Noah after the flood, we are told that God spoke to Noah and said: 'Behold, I establish my covenant with you and your offspring after you, and with every living creature that is with you, the birds, the livestock, and every beast of the earth with you, as many as came out of the ark, it is for every beast of the earth' (Gen. 9.8–10).

Likewise, according to the Pauline letters in the New Testament, we are the creatures with whom God united himself in the Incarnation and became man. And this was in order to 'unite all things in him, things in heaven and things on earth' (Eph. 1.10) and 'to reconcile to himself all things, whether on earth or in heaven' (Col. 1.19–20). Here, as in the Old Testament, it is made clear that the beasts living with man on earth enter through us into a special relationship with God. Thus on a Christian understanding, it is our role and responsibility as covenanted stewards of creation to include the animals in our care for ourselves, especially as the animals and the whole of creation is said to be crying out for salvation (cf., Rom. 8.18–25).

It is true that this understanding of the biblical teaching about our relationship with animals before God is quite different from that sometimes attributed to Thomas Aquinas, whom even fellow Christians have accused of promoting an instrumental attitude to animals.[3] It is also true that St Thomas said, with reference to Aristotle's *Politics*, that 'it is not unlawful to use plants for the good of animals and animals for the good of man' (ST, I, II, q. 64). And when he spoke of using animals he certainly meant that we have a right to kill them for food. He wrote:

> Now the most necessary use would seem to consist in the fact that animals use plants, and men use animals, for food, and this cannot be done unless these be deprived of life; wherefore it is lawful both to take life from plants for the use of animals, and from animals for the use of men. In fact this is in keeping with the commandment of God Himself: for it is written (Gn 1:29–30): 'Behold I have given you every herb . . . and all the trees . . . to be your meat, and to all beasts of the earth' and again (Gn 9:3): 'Everything that moveth and liveth shall be meat to you'.
> (ST, I, II, q. 64)

But while he refers to the animals as a necessary source of food, nowhere does St Thomas say that we may abuse animals. Moreover, his reference to Genesis 9 implies that he sees the eating of meat as a special concession granted to humans in an imperfect world. In a perfect world things would be different.

Much the same position is adopted by the Swiss Reformist theologian Karl Barth. As he notes, not only is there no reference to the killing of animals for food in Genesis 1, which speaks of the beginning and a world free of sin, but there are also many biblical references to the end of this world which depict a world in which there is again total peace between all creatures, and so no animal slaughter (Barth, 1961: 353). The prophet Isaiah speaks of a time when 'the wolf shall lie down with lamb' (Isa. 11.6) and of the 'lion eating straw like the ox' (Isa. 65.25). And acting as the mouthpiece of God, Hosea says: 'And I will make for them a covenant on that day with the beasts of the field and the birds of the heavens, and the creeping things on the ground. And I will abolish the bow, the sword, and war from the land, and I will make you lie down in safety' (Hos. 2.18). Commenting on this Barth writes:

> The history of the creature fashioned by the Word of God begins with the great episode in which the peace between God and itself is broken by man. The interim period which follows is the only time when the peace between creature and creature is broken and replaced by the struggle for existence. Only now can the animal become the enemy, disturber and destroyer of man and *vice versa*. Creation and consummation are the boundaries of history, and therefore of this interim period, and therefore of the time when man's lordship over the animal can and must also mean that the animal threatens man and that man slays the animal in order to live. (Barth, 1961: 355)

According to Barth, while ours is the world described as 'interim', we must have good reasons for killing animals. That man has been given a dispensation by God also means that he cannot kill animals just because he wants to. Doing so, Barth suggests, would be akin to murder (Barth, 1961: 355). Man is responsible before God for the way he uses and kills animals. He must show pity and inflict as little pain and suffering as possible. Even as a killer must the human act as a friend of the animal. Speaking of hunting, slaughter and vivisection, Barth says that in these contexts, 'if anywhere, animal protection, care and friendship are quite indispensable' (Barth, 1961: 355).

Similarly, the Catechism of the Catholic Church, while reminding us of the gentleness with which saints like St Francis of Assisi treated animals, also declares that it 'it is legitimate to use animals for food and clothing' and that 'medical and scientific experimentation on animals is a morally acceptable practice if it remains within reasonable limits and contributes to caring for or saving human lives' (*Catechism*, para. 2417). It warns, however, that 'it is contrary to human dignity to cause animals to suffer or die needlessly' (*Catechism*, para. 2418).

Having shown that it is not true that traditional Christian teachings have expressed scant respect for animals and have imparted an instrumental attitude towards animals, we may take note of Scott Bader-Saye's observation that 'a failure to exercise virtuous dominion over the non-human animals will lead to the distortion of human character and a clouding of the divine image' (Bader-Saye, 2001: 7), that is, a clouding of our likeness to a God of love and care.

SHOULD WE BE VEGETARIANS?

Does the use of animals for food partly spoil our image of a loving God? Perhaps we should seek to realize a world in which the lamb can lie down with the wolf, or a world in which we do not eat animals or deprive them of life for any other reason? Well, most of us are meat eaters. Most cultures, and most religions, allow the killing and eating of animals, or at least certain kinds of animal, although the regulations regarding slaughter vary between different cultures and religions. It is also true, however, that there are many believers as well as unbelievers who are vegetarian on grounds of conscience. Bader-Saye – a Christian – suggests that vegetarianism reflects a morally sounder attitude towards animals than meateating. He writes:

> Perhaps if we come to understand the *imago Dei* not primarily as the conferring of privilege or status but as an election of humans for the service and care of the other creatures, we would begin also to re-envision our practices of meat-eating, experimentation and the harvesting of animals.   (Bader-Saye, 2001: 12–13)

And Singer – an atheist – suggests that there is arrogance in eating meat. In his view, not only does meat eating reflect an attitude of superiority towards animals, but it also shows that 'we regard their life and well-being subordinate to our taste for a particular kind of dish' (Singer, 1989: 79). He says that 'our practice of rearing and killing other animals in order to eat them is a clear instance of the sacrifice of the most important interests of other beings in order to satisfy trivial interests of our own' (Singer, 1989: 79). He says 'trivial' because he holds that there is no nutritional advantage in meat-eating compared with a balanced vegetarian diet. In short, to his mind, we have a moral obligation to cease the practice of eating meat.

Whether or not all experts on nutrition would agree with Singer, on a Judaeo-Christian understanding, we have, as noted, been granted a divine dispensation to use animals for food. But this, as Barth observed, is with a proviso. We are not supposed to cause unnecessary pain and suffering when slaughtering animals. Is the Barthian position reasonable?

Most of us seem to think so. And so UK and EU law, which allow the killing of animals for meat production, state that animals should be slaughtered as humanely as possible. According to the Directive 93/119/EC On the Protection of Animals at the Time of Slaughter or Killing – which was implemented in the UK by the Welfare of Animals (Slaughter or Killing) Regulations 1995 – it is an offence to cause or permit an animal avoidable excitement, pain and suffering.[4] Thus UK slaughterhouses are monitored by the Food Standards Agency, while the killing of animals on farms or 'knackers' yards is monitored by the State Veterinary Service. And mostly it is normal practice to stun animals before killing them, though special provision is provided for Jews and Muslims whose religions require them to bleed animals. It should be noted, however, that according to a 1999 amendment to the 1995 Act, religious slaughter can only be carried out in approved slaughter houses.

These regulations reflect the view that it is morally acceptable to breed and kill animals for food, provided the animals are slaughtered in a humane way to avoid suffering.

SO HOW SHOULD WE NOT TREAT FARM ANIMALS?

The UK was one of the first countries in the world to introduce laws to protect farm animals. This was with the Protection of Animals

Act 1911, an Act which has since been amended numerous times in keeping with the times. Today, under the Protection of Animals Acts 1911–2000, it is an offence to cause unnecessary suffering to any domestic or captive animal by means such as cruel beating, overloading or inhumane conditions of transport. Moreover, it is forbidden to take part in the fighting or baiting of any animal. Cock fighting has long been forbidden under a special Act, namely the Cock Fighting Act 1952. Furthermore, the system of keeping calves closely confined in veal crates has been banned in the UK since 1990. And it may be added that in January 2007 it was banned within the whole of the EU – largely thanks to the campaigning organization *Compassion in World Farming* (CWF).

This does not mean, however, that all is well and that all farm animals have a wonderful life. A few examples to the contrary will suffice to prove the point. Veal is still being produced in the UK. And while the calves are no longer kept in veal crates, they are still kept in narrowly confined spaces. Indeed, the Welfare of Farm Animals (England) Regulations 2000, allow a person to keep a calf in a single pen provided the calf is free to turn around without difficulty, and the width of the pen or stall is not less than the height of the calf at the withers. Other practices affecting young cattle include castration. This should always be carried out under an anaesthetic, but it would appear that there is a certain amount of malpractice. The practice of removing calves from their mothers at the age of two or three days might also be described as cruel, cruel to the calves and cruel to the cows. Yet such is the fate of many factory-farmed dairy cows and their calves.

If calves often have a raw deal, the same is no less true of broiler and factory-farmed egg-laying chickens. The practice of trimming the beaks on battery egg-laying chickens is still allowed in the UK, as well as in most other European states, though a ban will be introduced under EU law in 2011. The practice of beak trimming is undertaken to avoid harmful pecking, which would otherwise be a problem in the crammed conditions under which the battery chickens live. That may well seem a good reason for the practice. But beak trimming is a painful procedure. It involves cutting through bone, cartilage and soft tissue.

Broiler chickens may be better off than their egg-laying cousins. This is because they are not raised in cages. They are, however, often housed in cramped, dark and hot sheds. There is little doubt that, in the world of farmed poultry, free-range chickens have the best life. If they are locked up, they are, at least, locked up in big spaces.

If factory farming is cruel towards animals, it also entails risks for humans. This is because factory farming involves confining great numbers of animals to crammed spaces. To be sure, factory farming, which today is found in most parts of the world, provides the ideal conditions for spreading infections and for the development of new more virulent mutations of both viruses and bacteria.

Indeed, it may be noted that an editorial published in April 2006 in the UK's leading medical journal, *The Lancet*, put forward the view that there are strong grounds for holding factory farming responsible for the highly pathogenic strain of bird flu virus H5N1, which is posing a global threat to man and beast. In other words, it was argued that it is wrong to suggest that wild birds are the main portents of bird flu and that 'far more likely to be perpetuating the spread of the virus is the movement of poultry, poultry products or infected material from poultry farms' (*The Lancet*, vol. 6, 8 April, 2006: x).

In agreement with this argument, the Green Party Euro MP Caroline Lucas, in her report, *Avian Influenza: Time to Shut the Intensive Poultry 'Flu Factories?*, published in July 2006, called for an outright ban on factory farming as a way of preventing the further spread of the deadly H5N1 strain of bird flu (Lucas, 2006). She also appealed to the WHO to recommend free-range farming and that birds should be kept outside wherever possible. Furthermore, she said that the EU should halt all imports and exports of live poultry and hatching eggs and make permanent its ban on cross-border trade in wild birds.

The argument for the view that factory farming is responsible for the H5N1 strain of avian flu is also supported by GRAIN, an international non-governmental organization promoting sustainable farm management and agricultural biodiversity. This organization too points a finger at Southeast Asian poultry factory farming, which has snowballed over the last few decades.[5] Like the *Lancet* editorial, GRAIN espouses the opinion that wild birds are unlikely to spread the deadly bird flu, because very few wild birds have been found to be infected with the H5N1 virus. The organization points out that 'nearly all wild birds that have tested positive for the disease were dead and, in most cases, found near outbreaks in domestic poultry'. On this line of argument, wild birds have been infected with the deadly H5N1 bird flu strain by domestic birds, and not the other way round!

HUNTING

In the face of fierce protests by its supporters, fox-hunting was banned in England and Wales during 2005, having been enjoyed as a sport for centuries. Linked to horse riding and point-to-points it is for some a much loved rural tradition. Indeed, the ban was seen as a slap in the face by many rural dwellers, who in support of the sport argued that there are too many foxes, which if true would be a good reason for reducing the numbers of these animals. The supporters of fox-hunting also deny that it is unnecessarily cruel. They say it is in keeping with nature's ways.

But it was precisely because it was seen as cruel that it was banned. Opponents of the sport argue that there are other more humane ways of killing foxes. They say that hunting foxes with hounds is barbaric, because when the hounds catch the foxes, they tear the tired animals apart after having chased them for miles through field after field. This suggests that some of those who oppose fox-hunting might be in favour of other types of hunting. Some might accept hunting involving the direct shooting and killing of the animal. So, is hunting acceptable as a sport, provided it involves as little suffering as possible on the part of the hunted animal? And what about hunting, not as a sport, but as a means of feeding ourselves?

Andrew Linzey argues that it is not only the means of killing and the suffering inflicted that count, but also human attitudes. He says that fox-hunting 'is not undertaken (as killing should be) as a regrettable act sometimes made necessary in a sinful and fallen world, rather it is celebrated as a "sport"' (Linzey, 2002b). On this line of reasoning, hunting as a sport, hunting for fun, is not acceptable. It is seen as wanton killing merely for pleasure, whereas hunting to survive could be justified. That is, hunting to feed ourselves could be justified.

To be sure, hunting is older than agriculture. Mankind has hunted since time immemorial to provide food for tribe and family. Clearly there is no more reason to object to hunting or fishing for food than there is to disagree with animal farming for food. If we allow animal farming, we can have no objection to hunting and fishing for food, provided it is not undertaken in a cruel way or in a way that threatens biodiversity and the environment and in the end even our own food supply. On the contrary, hunting is arguably preferable to animal breeding inasmuch as the animals are left living in the wild free to pursue their natural habits.

As noted, hunting also seems justified as a way of keeping the populations of certain kinds of animal under control and making sure that they do not become an environmental threat. It may even be a way of making sure that there is no shortage of food for them. However, it might be added that this does not mean that those who hunt for these kinds of reason might not also see hunting as a sport and enjoy it. But is it wrong to take pleasure in hunting if the activity can be justified on other grounds? Surely what is wrong is killing just for the pleasure of killing.

ANIMAL EXPERIMENTATION

As we have seen in Chapter 9, in Article 5 of the Helsinki Declaration, adopted by the World Medical Association in 1964, it is stated that: 'In research on man, the interest of science and society should never take precedence over considerations related to the well-being of the subject'. According to Linzey, this statement, which relates to adults and children, should be extended to embrace unborn humans and also animals. In Linzey's view, 'the subjugation of any being, human, foetal or animal to experimental procedures against its own interest must be morally wrong' (Linzey, 1987: 139).

However, if we agree with the widely accepted assumption that human lives are worth more than animal lives, we are justified in using animals in medical research for the sake of saving human lives when there is no alternative way of gaining the information sought and provided we seek to minimize the suffering of the animal. Is this unreasonable? As we have seen, on a Christian understanding, the answer is 'no'. However, not even a utilitarian like Singer says no to all animal experimentation. This may seem to contradict his statement that animals should be given the same consideration as humans. However, as he declared when interviewed on a BBC 2 programme, *Monkeys, Rats and Me: Animal Testing*, screened on 18 February 2007, some animal research is justifiable in terms of the immense good it may bring about for mankind. Surely, most of us would agree. It may be added that we should not forget that some animal research, such as research into vaccine against animal diseases, is for the benefit of animals.

One might ask, however, whether Singer's position is reasonable, given that he is a utilitarian opposed to specism. The answer is that his position is far from unreasonable. There are good utilitarian grounds for affording us humans a special status with reference to our ability to suffer. We are capable of suffering not only from what has happened or is happening to us, be it psychologically or physiologically painful for us, but we are also capable of psychological suffering in anticipation of future suffering. Even if some animals, such as the apes, to some extent may share this ability, we humans are certainly more self-aware and intelligent than animals. On utilitarian lines of reasoning, this should make for an important difference between us and animals, one that is morally relevant, one that provides a reason to afford us preferential treatment. If we are capable of more and of different psychological suffering, our suffering should be given greater weight than that of animals. Hence, on utilitarian as well as on Judaeo-Christian lines of reasoning, we might allow ourselves to use animals to promote human health and wellbeing, provided we do not inflict needless or excessive suffering on animals.

Benefits and drawbacks

So how might animal experiments benefit humans – and, indeed, other animals? The UK organization RDS, Understanding Animal Research in Medicine (formerly known as Research Defense Society), which represents medical researchers in the public debate, presents a number of arguments for the use of animals in medical research. They point to a long list of medical advances made possible only because of such research. Among the developments mentioned are: blood transfusions in the 1910s, the first modern anaesthetics in the 1920s, broad spectrum antibiotics in the late 1930s, a number of different vaccines in the 1940s and 1950s, chemotherapy in the 1960s, efficient drugs to control transplant rejection, new drugs to treat viral diseases in the 1980s; and combined drugs therapies to control HIV infection in the 1990s.[6] The list is impressive and represents a strong argument in favour of animal testing of medical products and procedures. In fact, most modern drugs, vaccines, anaesthetics and surgical techniques have been tested on animals before being tried on humans. And no new drug can be tested on humans in the UK, unless it has first been tested on two different kinds of animal, one of which must be a large non-rodent (UK Medicines Act 1968).

It is, however, clear that it is desirable to minimize the use of animal experiments, to use as few animals as possible and to consider alternative testing methods where available. And surely, when animals are used, as few animals as possible should be used. Animals are sentient creatures. This, as argued, makes it wrong to inflict unnecessary pain on them. It is therefore a welcome development that today nearly all animal testing is undertaken for medical reasons, as opposed to more trivial reasons. At least this is true in the UK where animal testing for cosmetics is no longer allowed, although under UK law it is still permitted to use animals to test the safety of agricultural products, industrial chemicals and household cleaning products.

If the suffering inflicted on animals is an important consideration, so too is another seldom mentioned aspect of animal research. This is, as Bader-Saye has pointed out, the dulling effect it may have on the researcher. C. S. Lewis too warned us about this when he said that 'if, on the basis of mere preference for those like ourselves, we say that we can undertake cruel experiments on animals, then we might find that on the very same basis we come to the conclusion that we can undertake painful or degrading experiments on certain categories of humans' (Lewis, 1989: 597–8).

Not only are the moral aspects and the possible psychological consequences of animal research important, but there are also medical or scientific considerations to be taken into account. Animals are biologically different from humans. Therefore, as noted in Chapter 8, the effects of drugs and toxins on animals may differ from the effects on humans. There have been cases when drugs have had no adverse effects on tested animals but have had disastrous consequences when subsequently tested on humans. Since tests on animals can be misleading, it should always be asked whether the testing really would be helpful and therefore really is necessary. That is, the UK requirement that all drugs should first be tested on animals is arguably scientifically unsound.

Practice and regulations

In the UK medical research involving animals is regulated under the Animals (Scientific Procedures) Act 1986, a stringent piece of animal-research legislation.[7] It stipulates that animals should be used only when the research in question cannot be undertaken using other methods, that the minimal number of animals should be used and also that the discomfort and suffering of animals be kept to a minimum with the appropriate use of anaesthetics and pain killers.

As for the kinds of animal used in research, over 80 per cent of animals in the UK are rodents, usually rats and mice, while research using cats, dogs and horses accounts for less than 1 per cent of animal experiments and is only undertaken if other species are unsuitable. And it may be noted that apes, that is gorillas, chimpanzees and orang-utans, have not been used in the UK for over 20 years. This is because they are threatened species and also because they are thought to suffer acutely from being kept in a laboratory environment. As to monkeys they are less fortunate. They are used in some 0.15 per cent of experiments, which might sound like a small percentage. But in real numbers it means that every year thousands of monkey experiments take place in the UK. For Home Office figures show that each year some 3 million animals are used in research in this country.

Indeed, the Home Office figures raise questions about current efforts to reduce the number of animals used. In May 2004 the British government created a new body, The National Centre for the Replacement, Refinement and Reduction of Animals (NC3Rs), to advocate and advise on animal alternatives. The first of the three Rs, 'Replacement', stands for the search for alternatives to the use of animals. Among alternatives to animal experiments and testing are test-tube studies on human cell and tissue cultures, including laboratory grown skin tissue. Computer models and statistics are also used. In addition, it is possible to give human subjects drug doses too small to trigger adverse reactions, but big enough for their effects to be assessed by examination of the subject's blood plasma. This is called micro-dosing. It would, however, appear that efforts to reduce the number of animals used in research have failed. Even if overall fewer animals are used in research today than earlier, many animals are used more than once. In addition, there has been an increased demand for genetically modified (GM) animals. According to the Royal Society, today 21 per cent of animals used in research are GM animals, which are used to study the function of specific genes and the development of human diseases.

The second R, 'Refinement', stands for efforts to reduce the distress and suffering of animals used in medical experiments. This involves the development and encouragement of the use of anaesthetics and pain killers as well as the use of lower doses when chemicals are being tested for their safety. The aim of the third R, 'Reduction', is to use as few animals as possible for each experiment or on each testing occasion and thus waste the lives of as few animals as possible. This aim, like the first, may be promoted with the help of statistics and new technologies.

While the success in implementing the three Rs may have been no more than partial, the initiative bears witness to an increasing awareness of our responsibility not to inflict needless suffering on animals. Sometimes, this awareness does, however, take exaggerated forms. Several groups who are actively protesting against animal experimentation have resorted to violent means. On the understanding that violence fosters violence, this can only be counter-productive. Arguments for a total ban on the use of animals in medical research and for safety testing may deserve a hearing, but not by means of threats and intimidation.

CONCLUSION

Talk about animal rights is not unreasonable if by this we mean that their rights are constituted by our obligations towards them. That we do have obligations towards them is, as shown, widely recognized. It is recognized in the many laws and regulations stipulating how we should and should not treat animals. And it is recognized in Judaeo-Christian views on our relationship to animals. What is less widely accepted is the understanding that it is wrong to eat meat. This view is neither endorsed within the Judaeo-Christian tradition in the West nor within the Muslim religion, nor is it sanctioned in secular law. Indeed, within most, if not all, societies humans are allowed to use animals, or at least certain animals, for food. We are allowed to do so, but should avoid cruel means of slaughter and cruel farming practices. Given our obligations towards animals not to inflict needless suffering, certain farming practices must be described as controversial, as is hunting merely for the pleasure of killing. Given our obligation not to inflict needless suffering on animals, it also follows that animal research should be restricted as far as possible and only used as a last resort to test new medical products or procedures. Wanton cruelty and unnecessary destruction of animal life can never be justified.

CHAPTER 11

ECOLOGY AND THE GUARDIANS OF CREATION

When I look at the heavens, the work of your fingers, the moon and
the stars, which you have set in place,
What is man that you are mindful of him, and the son of man that you
care for him?
Yet you have made him a little lower than the heavenly beings, and
crowned him with glory and honour.
You have given him dominion over the works of your hands; you have
put all things under his feet, all sheep and oxen, and also all the beasts
of the field, the birds of the heavens, and the fish of the sea, whatever
passes along the paths of the seas.

Ps. 8.3–8

INTRODUCTION: THE HUMAN FOOTPRINT

The Psalmist talks about the wonders of the world, noting that our
position is unique and emphasizing our role as caretakers. The world
is said to be in human hands. But he does not say that we own the
world. Not, then, as owners but as stewards have we humans a
special responsibility to care for the world, as what we do and fail to
do make a difference not only to us here and now but also to other
creatures and for the future. Planet Earth travels towards its future
with humankind at the helm. Our powers may be limited, but we are
the pilots on whom the other passengers depend.

Thus as the prophet Hosea says, when we act without foresight
and merely to satisfy our own gratification, 'the country is mourn-
ing, and all who live in it pine away, even the wild animals and the
birds in heaven, the fish of the sea themselves are perishing' (Hos.
4.3). The wisdom of Hosea is plain.[1] The soil we till is a gift to be

cherished with humility and gratitude. It is there not only for us but also for other life forms together with which we share this planet, on whose good health all earthly life depends.

Today more than ever human action is setting its stamp on the world. Our footprints are everywhere. Our technologies have done much to improve the existence for humankind. But it is also true that our technologies are affecting the world by polluting the seas and the atmosphere. With our technologies we are changing the world not only for ourselves and for future human generations but also for other creatures. Our sprawling cities as well as our agriculture, our reservoirs and dams, our fishing and our forestry, not only affect our own species, but these things have an impact on the whole earthly biosphere, present and future.

We are an integral part of the ecosystem. What we do affects all life forms. And so, what we do to the environment affects not least ourselves. For 'we ourselves are part of creation, formed out of the earth, and dependent on the rest of creation for our continued existence . . . caring for creation is part of caring for ourselves' (Catholic Bishops' Conference of England and Wales, 2002: 7).

Calling for sustainable management of natural resources and for economic policies allowing 'men, women and children to flourish along with all the diversity of creation' (Berry, 2000: 21), the authors of the *Evangelical Declaration on the Care of Creation*, of 1994, say that 'the earthly result of human sin has been a perverted stewardship, a patchwork of garden and wasteland in which the waste is increasing' (Berry, 2000: 20). Thus if mankind has used and abused creation in shortsighted and selfish ways by land and water degradation, deforestation and ruthless species extinction, the time has come to work vigorously to protect and heal creation or, if that is not possible, to alleviate the symptoms of ecological damage. In short, the message is: do not steal from the future to give to the present.

This chapter, which deals with ecological issues such as those pointed to above, starts with a discussion of what might be described as unnatural ways of farming and wasteful uses or abuses of natural resources such as forests and seas. But not only is it important not to exhaust natural resources. Our biggest ecological concern today must be that of climate change. This therefore is the issue with which the second and larger part of this chapter is concerned. And in this context we will consider the Gaia theory, according to which the global climate is as dependent on life on Earth as life on Earth is on the climate.

SOME ECOLOGICAL CONCERNS

Deep ecologists, who identify themselves with nature and other creatures, are not alone in advocating caution with respect to the use of herbicides, insecticides and other chemicals. Nor are they alone in urging caution when cutting down forests and trawling the seas. Most of us are aware of a number of warning examples illustrating the inadvisability of certain activities.

The BSE (mad-cow disease) epidemic among British cattle is a striking example of what might go wrong. First confirmed in 1986, it is believed to have been spread by cattle fed on meat-and-bone meal made from BSE-infected brain tissue. The disease is related to scrapie, which is found in sheep and goats, as well as to Creutzfeld-Jacob disease (CJD), which is a fatal form of dementia affecting humans. All three diseases are Transmissible Spongiform Encephalopathies (TSEs) resulting from the build-up of abnormal prion proteins in the brain and nervous system.

In 1996 a new strain of CJD was discovered in the UK. Found especially among people in areas where there had been a high incidence of BSE, this new strain was believed to be caused by eating meat from BSE infected cattle. This led to the introduction of a number of precautionary measures to protect humans. Thousands of animals were slaughtered. And to avoid further transmission of the disease among grazing animals, the practice of giving animal feed to ruminants was banned in 1988. In addition, those parts of cattle, sheep and goats that could be BSE-infected now have to be removed when an animal is slaughtered. The reason for the application of these laws not only to cattle is that BSE was later found to be prevalent also among sheep and goats.

More recently, a new strain of MRSA has been reported among farmers in the Netherlands, Belgium and Denmark. Resistant to most commonly used antibiotics and causing skin, heart and bone infections, it is suspected that this new strain first arose in pigs fed antibiotics and that it then spread from pigs to humans. If this is correct, it shows how excessive use of antibiotics, be it in animals or humans, may lead to drug-resistant strains of bacteria. In other words, this new strain of MRSA is noteworthy, because the increasing number of drug resistant strains of bacteria is a major cause of concern today.

Another cause of concern is the use of chemicals such as oestrogen-like compounds derived from various types of pesticides, including DDT. There are many reports about the gender-bending effects on bird and fish of these types of chemical. Nor are they safe for humans. DDT is considered particularly harmful. Nonetheless, although it is banned in the EU, DDT is still used in some parts of Africa to combat the malaria mosquito.

Are scientists, biotechnology companies and politicians throwing caution to the wind for the sake of short-term gains?

One much debated issue, and one that has put the EU at odds with the USA, is that of genetically modified (GM) food products. Since 1998 the import of most types of GM food from the USA and countries such as Argentina and Canada has effectively been banned within the EU. This is because of warnings to the effect that some varieties of GM food could have adverse effects on human health. Concerns have also been voiced about the possibility that GM crops might contaminate the environment. There are fears about cross-breeding with conventional varieties and that GM plants may act as invasive intruders taking over neighbouring fields.

The UK has, however, long been leading a campaign to ease restrictions and open up European markets to GM food. This is on the ground that there have actually been no reports about negative effects on the environment or about adverse side-effects in humans linked to GM produce. For example, years of farming trials have produced no scientific reports of adverse environmental effects of the cultivation of GM maize. Rather, the opposite seems to be the case. To be sure, it is clear that some GM crops might have advantages over conventional varieties. They might be more pest resistant. They could be modified to withstand drought or to thrive in salty soil where conventional varieties would fare poorly. There is no doubt that GM food has a potential to save thousands, if not millions, from hunger.

But whether such hopes will be realized depends not only on the enhanced resistance and yields of GM crops, but also on politicians and biotechnology companies. Big biotechnology companies, such as Monsanto, are geared to profit-making. It has been argued that some of their policies are to the disadvantage of their customers. One such policy is Monsanto's sale of high-yielding cereal varieties that self-destruct after one generation. This kind of cereal does not allow farmers to re-sow year after year but forces them to buy new seed for sowing each year. This, then, is a policy that may disadvantage poor farmers, especially those in the developing world. Thus even if GM crops could have many advantages, there are several reasons why many people are sceptical about them.

Indeed, at the same time as the biotechnology industry is trying to produce new types of genetically engineered products, there is an increasing trend towards organic farming. This is not only in Europe. This trend is also visible in Canada, one of the main producers of GM food together with the USA, Argentina and Brazil. More interesting still, this trend is driven by consumer demand. The greening of the public is also taking other forms such as recycling and a preference for local produce to reduce the climatic effects of long-distance transport.

It would seem that there is an increasing awareness that when man no longer acts as a humble steward and treads lightly on the soil he tills, but like a Prometheus arrogates to himself any powers he can, he becomes a danger to himself and others. Thus today it is not only intergovernmental organizations such as the United Nations that are calling for action to promote green policies for the sake of human health, the health of other species and the health of our planet. There is a public awareness which is reflected in widespread support for non-governmental bodies such as Greenpeace, Friends of the Earth and the WWF. Groups such as these argue not only for the protection of natural resources seen as human consumables, but according to their philosophy, the biodiversity and beauty of the world are also riches of intrinsic value. And so they work for the protection of endangered animal species as well as for human welfare when promoting sustainable management of forests, freshwater and marine areas.

They argue that measures such as good forest management both promote wildlife and natural beauty and also help populations in countries ranging from Nepal, to Uganda and India, Costa Rica and China by protecting their means of living. Of course, many people in tropical areas live off the forest, just as many people close to the sea live off the sea. For both types of population it is important to sustain the natural resources that they rely on for food and income. That exploitation which threatens animal habitats and natural resources may also threaten man is especially true in the case of the tropical rain forests and the seas.

The rain forests contain an enormous amount of animal and plant species. And it is noteworthy that most of the nutrients supporting the rich variety of life in these forests are found in the plants rather than in the soil. Many of the tree-climbing plants do not take their water from the ground but directly from rainwater. This means that if you cut down the trees, you also lose much of the nutrients and physical support of other life forms. All you may be left with is barren soil.

Tropical hardwood is, however, valuable on the commercial market. This provides a temptation to cut trees down for short-term profit. Of concern too is the clearing of tropical forests to convert them into various types of plantation for short-term gain. This applies even to plantations of bio-fuels. Today both humans and other species, such as African gorillas, chimpanzees and bonobos, are increasingly threatened by activities such as these. So too are the Asian elephant, the Sumatran tiger and the Borneo orang-utan.

Moreover, not only are the forests, and in particular the rain-forests, important habitats for indigenous species and a means of income for local people, but these ecosystems also help to stabilize the global climate. This is especially true of the tropical rainforests, which absorb and store large amounts of carbon dioxide, too much of which promotes global warming.

The creation of national parks and conservancies which are actively managed may be part of the answer in a world threatened by deforestation. It would allow forests to thrive and let animal populations increase with benefits to local communities as well as to global climate. Uganda's national park with its mountain gorillas is an example of an economic asset to people living in surrounding areas. Moreover, it helps us all by preserving an ecological niche important for climate regulation.

No less important than the forests, the seas too regulate the climate. Ocean algae, like tropical forests, absorb atmospheric carbon dioxide and so influence the climate. The seas are also the source of rain, so necessary for life. In addition, seas, lakes and rivers are important sources of human food.

But today over-fishing and water pollution pose major threats. Waste is building up at the bottom of seas as sewage and other leftovers are being dumped. Heavy metals are polluting our oceans and entering the food chain. Rivers are being poisoned by pesticides and other chemicals. Oil spills are spoiling beaches and causing harm to fish and birds. Many fish species are at risk of extinction because of industrial fishing. According to the United Nations, rising demand for seafood and other marine produce is set to lead to a collapse of today's commercial fish stocks by 2050 unless better management is introduced (UN Press Report, 5 February 2007). Not only are we over-fishing, but we are fishing in destructive ways. Bottom trawling using enormously long nets is wasteful. Much of the catch is thrown back into the sea. Among this waste are small crabs, sponges, corals and even fish. Commercial whaling is another concern. It has reduced today's whale population to a fraction of what it was a century ago.

We are at risk of depleting the seas of many of its riches. Both governments and individual communities need to show restraint and implement green policies to preserve what is one of our greatest assets of all.

IS GLOBAL WARMING MAN-MADE?

The Intergovernmental Panel on Climate Change (IPCC) leaves us in no doubt that human emissions of carbon dioxide and other so-called greenhouse gases are playing a major role in climate change. Thus the IPCC, which was established in 1988 by the World Meteorological Organization (WMO) and the United Nations Environmental Programme (UNEP), tells us that climate change is not a future problem. It is a problem that must be tackled now. Based on computer models and actual climate observations, IPPC studies, representing the work of several hundred scientific experts, show that global warming is a fact: 'Warming of the climate is unequivocal, as is now evident from observations of increases in global air and ocean temperatures, widespread melting of snow and ice, rising global sea levels' (IPCC, 1, 2007: 5).

Indeed, IPCC statistics speak for themselves. Eleven of the last twelve years, from 1995 to 2006, rank among the twelve warmest years ever recorded. That is, they are the warmest since 1850 when the World Meteorological Organization's records began (IPCC, I, 2007: 5). Not only that, but average northern hemisphere temperatures during the second half of the twentieth century were most likely higher than during any other 50-year period in the last 500 years and probably the highest in the past 1,300 years. Moreover, the last time the polar areas were significantly warmer than at present for an extended period of time was about 125,000 years ago. And then reductions in polar ice volumes led to a 4–6 metres sea level rise (IPCC, I, 2007: 10).

Extreme too were the global temperatures in the year 2006. From a global perspective, 2006 was the sixth warmest year on record according to the World Meteorological Organization. It may be noted that the year 2006 was also the warmest year ever recoded in the UK, where records date back to 1659. Then, in the summer of 2007, the UK witnessed a rain record that led to flooding in large parts of central England. This too may be attributable to climate change.

That the remarkable rise in global temperatures has gone hand in hand with increasing emissions of greenhouse gases, above all carbon dioxide, is beyond dispute. Today our atmosphere is very different from that in pre-industrial times, which strongly suggests that global warming is largely man-made.

> Global atmospheric concentrations of carbon dioxide, methane and nitrous oxide have increased markedly as a result of human activities since 1750 and now far exceed pre-industrial values determined from ice cores spanning many thousand years. The global increases in carbon dioxide concentration are due primarily to fossil fuel use and land-use change, while those of methane and nitrous oxide are primarily due to agriculture.
>
> (IPCC, I, 2007: 2)

The main culprit is carbon dioxide. Indeed, over the last ten years carbon dioxide concentrations have increased even faster than earlier predicted, mainly as a result of the burning of fossil fuels by electric power plants, industry, cars and household heating.

EFFECTS OF GLOBAL WARMING

The IPCC has made predictions about how climate change of up to 5 °C would affect us globally. Based partly on observed temperature increases between 1990 and 2005 and on projections relating to global greenhouse gas emissions, it is estimated that 'continued greenhouse emissions at or above current rates would cause further warming and induce many changes in the global climate system during the twenty-first century, changes that would very likely be larger than those observed during the twentieth century' (IPCC, I,

2007: 14). It is forecasted that this would be accompanied by a rise in sea levels of 28–44 cm by the end of the century, as Arctic and Antarctic ice masses melt. Indeed, an additional 10–20 cm is possible, if the recent dramatic melting of polar ice is continuing (IPCC, I, 2007: 7, 15). Other expected consequences of global warming are heat waves, tropical cyclones and heavy rainfalls. We might also witness a slowing down of the Gulf Stream, which would affect northern Europe by leading to a cooler rather than warmer climate (IPCC, I, 2007: 16).

But, on the assumption that the last mentioned scenario is not realized, climate change would mean that spring would come ever earlier to the north, which would affect 'leaf-unfolding, bird migration and egg-laying' and result in 'poleward and upward shifts in ranges in plant and animal species' worldwide (IPCC, II, 2007: 3). Agricultural crops would also have to be planted earlier. And heat waves might become more frequent and thus threaten millions in Europe and the USA. Another heat-related threat is malaria and other mosquito-borne diseases. If temperatures rise, disease-carrying mosquitoes might invade southern Europe and southern parts of the USA. Forest fires are another threat.

Some parts of the world would be more badly affected than others. Parts of Africa would suffer worse droughts than ever, leaving millions at risk of starving. With rising sea levels, some Pacific islands would sink into the seas. And low-lying coastal areas in other parts of the world, such as Bangladesh, would be at increased risk of flooding (IPCC, II, 2007: 4, 7, 8, 10). It is projected that by the end of the century millions of people will be flooded every year in densely populated low-lying areas increasingly affected by tropical storms.

To be sure, the poorest in the world would be the worst affected. Not only would growing seasons shrink in Africa due to droughts, but as the large lakes got smaller and warmer the fish population would decrease. Flooding and increased water temperatures in South, East and Southeast Asia would result in more cholera outbreaks and diarrhoeal disease. In parts of Latin America decreases in soil water are expected to lead to the replacement of tropical forest by savannah, while in other parts of the region salination of agricultural land might have an adverse effect on livestock and agriculture. Climate change will leave no part of the world unaffected (IPCC, II, 2007: 10–13). We are creating a different planet.

WHAT CAN WE DO?

The battle against climate change may be difficult, but, according to the IPCC, all may not yet be lost. Mankind has the know-how, if not the will, to stop global warming. With a concerted international effort, it would be possible to limit average global temperature rises within the next few decades to 2–3 °C. This is, however, not a likely scenario. More likely is a less ambitious programme, one that might curb a runaway rise in temperatures. To promote at least the last-mentioned scenario, the IPCC report suggests a number of measures which, if implemented, would limit global warming (IPCC, III, 2007: 1–21, 30–31):

- Nuclear energy – but it is admitted that 'safety, weapons and pro-liferation and waste remain constraints'.
- Renewable energy, such as electricity generated by windmills.
- Cleaner means of transport. The report suggests a 'shift from road to rail and inland waterway shipping', among other measures.
- Encouraging industries in both developed and developing countries to use clean energy.
- Energy efficient building materials both in industrial buildings and in private housing.
- Conservation of carbon stores, such as tropical forests, and 'financial incentives (national and international) to increase forest areas, reduce deforestation and maintain and manage forests'.
- Agricultural management involving efficient use of fertilizers and irrigation, reduction of emissions of methane and nitrous oxide.
- Waste management to reclaim energy.

It is noteworthy that the IPCC puts nuclear energy first on the list. This is noteworthy, because many environmentalists are worried about the disposal of harmful radioactive waste as well as about nuclear accidents such as that in Chernobyl in 1986. The Ukraine accident, which was the result of a flawed Soviet reactor-design, resulted in a number of deaths from burns and radiation. How many is unclear. It also caused fear, if not panic, about the consequences for wide areas of northern Europe exposed to nuclear fall-out.

Concerns such as these are real. So we should welcome UN statistics showing that the world is increasingly switching to clean and renewable power such as wind and solar energy (UN, *Trends in Sustainable Development*, 2007). That said, the UN statistics also show that, because of the industrialization of India and above all China, the consumption of fossil fuel is still growing. Indeed, the statistics tell us that, having overtaken the USA, China is now the world's biggest polluter.

GAIA AND DEEP ECOLOGY

As agents accountable before our children and our children's children, we have to do what we can to preserve the health of our planet. Our climate is in an unstable state. We are in an interglacial period. This alone makes for a lack of stability. And now we humans are adding to the instability.

According to James Lovelock, the well-known British scientist and originator of the Gaia theory, the Earth is a bio-system that has an intrinsic capacity to stay close to the right temperature and the right chemical composition for life. It has done so for over three billion years, a quarter of the time the universe has existed. Our planet is acting like a self-regulating organism. Plants and animals as well as dead matter interact, optimizing the conditions for life. We are dealing with a fine-tuned system that has maintained life-sustaining conditions for billions of years.

To Lovelock's mind, Gaia, the 'thin spherical shell of matter that surrounds the incandescent interior' of the Earth and which 'includes the biosphere and its dynamic physiological system' appears to have 'the unconscious goal of regulating the climate and the chemistry at a comfortable state for life' (Lovelock, 2006: 15). While Lovelock does not think that Gaia works according to a divine plan, he speaks of Gaia as if 'she' acts in a goal-directed manner. Lovelock would not say with the Psalmist that 'the Mighty One, God the Lord, speaks and summons the Earth from the rising of the sun to its setting' (Ps. 50.1). But he would say that Gaia works as an integrated unity to sustain life. 'The Earth System behaves as a single, self-regulating system comprised of physical, chemical, biological and human components', he says (Lovelock, 2006: 25).

How, then, exactly does Gaia work, as explained by Lovelock? Basically, 'she' works like this. The seas and the skies interact. Plant life, on land and in the seas, interacts with the atmosphere. Everything interacts. As noted above, oceanic algae pump down carbon dioxide from the atmosphere, as do tropical forests. This promotes life, since too much carbon dioxide makes for over-heating. Glaciers too help to avoid over-heating, since they reflect the sun's heat and thus send it back into the atmosphere. Moreover, marine organisms produce gases which, when oxidized in the air, produce cloud-condensation particles and thus make sure we have rain, which is needed for life on land. In addition, many animals eat plants, while plants are nourished by animal waste such as urea. Gaia, then, is the whole Earth system, 'organisms and material environment coupled together' (Lovelock, 2006: 23).

Although the sun has been getting hotter and hotter, life on Earth has survived. There have been ups and downs, yes. But Gaia has done remarkably well. 'Only for a very brief period in the Earth's history was the sun's warmth ideal for life, and that was about two billion years ago' (Lovelock, 2006: 44). Yet Gaia has managed to retain a relatively cool and comfortable temperature, one that favours life.

But today Gaia is facing an extraordinary challenge, as we humans are adding vast quantities of carbon dioxide and other greenhouse gases to the air. In addition, by cutting down rain forests capable of absorbing carbon dioxide, we are interfering with Gaia's temperature regulating system. This makes it doubly hard for Gaia to keep cool. The fact that Arctic ice is melting as a result of global warming promotes further global warming. Black soil and green moss reflect no heat back into space. Moreover, as sea temperatures rise, the seas will release trapped methane into the air, and methane is an even more potent greenhouse gas then carbon dioxide. In short, we are turning up the heat, while simultaneously removing the natural cooling-down systems. We are thus accelerating climate change.

The short-term remedy recommended by Lovelock for avoiding an escalating process running totally out of our control is nuclear energy until 'the energy that empowers the sun, and renewable energy are available' (Lovelock, 2006: 11). He is thus in agreement with the IPCC. To his mind, 'civilization is in imminent danger and has to use nuclear energy now, or suffer the pain soon to be inflicted by our out-raged planet' (Lovelock, 2006: 11). Lovelock also mentions the possibility of using space-mounted sunshades to cool the Earth by reflecting the sun's heat and sending it back into space. But he warns that technologies such as these should be regarded as short-term fixes doing no more than buying us time to change our damaging ways of life. In particular, he warns against making the earthly climate totally dependent on our interventions. Instead we should allow it to recuperate and regain its own balance and wellbeing.

> In the longer term we have to understand that however benign a technological solution may seem it has the potential to set humanity on a path to the ultimate form of slavery. The more we meddle with the Earth's composition and try to fix its climate, the more we take on the responsibility for keeping the Earth fit for life, until eventually our whole lives may be spent in drudgery doing the task that previously Gaia had freely done for over three billion years. This would be the worst of fates for us and reduce us to a truly miserable state, where we were forever wondering whether anyone, any nation or any international body, could be trusted to regulate the climate and the atmospheric composition. (Lovelock, 2006: 152)

Nonetheless, while warning us about putting too much trust in human technologies and governments, he says that he 'would like to see us use our technical skills to cure the ills of the Earth', much as a medical doctor seeks to cure his patients (Lovelock, 2006: 142).

While sharing a love and respect for nature with its proponents, Lovelock is no supporter of deep ecology. Coined by the Norwegian philosopher Arne Naess in the 1970s, the term deep ecology stands for a humanist philosophy and mysticism that scorns much of modern technology, urges us to live simple lives and involves a kind of self-identification with nature which entails that human life counts for no more than other life (Naess, 1978).

However, if Lovelock takes a more optimistic view of technology than deep ecologists, what his Gaia theory and their philosophy have in common is a holistic approach. That is to say, partly inspired by Gandhi's pacifism, Taoism and Buddhist philosophy, deep ecology is holistic in much the same way as the Gaia theory inasmuch as it is based on an understanding of the interconnectedness and interdependence not only of all life but also of life and lifeless nature. In addition, both Gaia theory and deep ecology reflect a kind of spirituality not foreign to religion. For as Ursula King writes:

> Conceptions of the world as a whole and of the organic unity of humankind – moreover, of the intrinsic unity of humankind and

the planet – are not alien to the religions of the world, for such universality of common belonging, of a shared origin and destiny, is often deeply enshrined in their original vision and teaching.

(King, 2006: 76)

The passage above by King is, however, not written with reference to either Lovelock or Naess, but with reference to the French twentieth-century Jesuit, palaeontologist and mystic Teilhard de Chardin, who, like Lovelock and Neass, had a holistic view of all earthly life as interrelated and an integral part of the biosphere as a whole. Teilhard expressed this view beautifully in *The Mass on the World*, a meditation dated 1923.

What my mind glimpsed through its hesitant explorations, what my heart craved with so little expectation of fulfilment, you now magnificently unfold for me: the fact that your creatures are not merely so linked together in solidarity that none can exist unless all the rest surround it, but that all are so dependent on a single central reality that a true life, borne in common by them all, gives them ultimately their consistence and their unity. (Teilhard, 1978: 124)

However, while Teilhard makes an implicit reference to God, neither Naess nor Lovelock is a Christian believer. Gaia may seem to work in a goal-directed manner, but on Lovelock's understanding, this is not because of divine design. His self-regulating Gaia has no need of God. Yet, interestingly, the Gaia theory leaves no room for the Darwinian understanding of evolution either. In terms of the Gaia theory, it is not only the case that the survival of various organisms is determined by external conditions, but it is also the case that external conditions are determined by the life-forms that are around. But according to Darwin's theory, what life-forms survive is totally dependent on surrounding conditions, including other surrounding organisms. Darwin's theory does not take into account the idea that external conditions such as climatic conditions are conditioned by the life-forms present. Moreover, and even more important, Darwin's world is one of brutal fight for life in a hostile environment. For him, as for Hobbes, organisms in the state of nature are in a constant fight against one another. Not so in the Gaia world. This is a world as much of mutual interplay and support as of competition. Here the very air we breathe depends as much on life as life depends on it.

Lovelock may think his theory has no need of God. But those of us who choose to believe, with Teilhard, that such a wonderful system of interdependence, so supportive of life, is to be explained with reference to divine providence need not think that the Gaia theory rules out the God hypothesis. The Gaia theory, according to which the Earth behaves as a self-regulating organism, is not incompatible with belief in God as the ultimate sustainer of life and director of the drama played out in space and time.

CONCLUSION

While we continue to exploit the world's natural resources and pollute the atmosphere, the soil and the seas, it is encouraging to note that there is an increasing environmental awareness, as witness both the work of the IPCC and various non-governmental organizations working for sustainable forestry, fishing and wildlife preservation and promoting the development of new and cleaner sources of energy. And it is encouraging to find that an attitude of reverence and gratitude for the natural beauty of this world and all its riches can be found among people of different faith and none, as can a sense of responsibility for what has been set before us. Indeed, today one senses an increasing awareness of our need to cherish, protect, preserve and care justly for the natural world, the world we all share, and share not only with other humans but also with creatures of other species. Increasingly, both those who see divine providence as part of the picture and those who leave God out of it seem to recognize the intrinsic interrelation of all life and realize that we humans have an important part to play in seeking to preserve an ecological balance that is hospitable towards life on Earth.

GLOSSARY

Abortifacient: an agent that produces an abortion

Adult stem cells: cells found in many tissues, e.g. bone marrow, that have the potential to form different types of cell

Amniotic fluid: fluid surrounding the foetus within the amniotic sac in the uterus

Amniocentesis: a prenatal test involving the removal of amniotic fluid

Animal-human chimeras: animals containing human cells added to them during early development

Blastocyst: an embryo 5–6 days after fertilization (if human)

Brain death: the cessation of brain function regulating breathing

Carrier testing: testing of adults to determine whether they risk passing on a genetic condition to their offspring

Chimera: an organism with two or more genetically distinct cell populations.

Chromosomes: the thread-like structures carrying the genes found in cell nuclei

Cloning: the production of a genetic copy of another organism (see Somatic Cell Nuclear Transfer (SCNT))

Conception: the union of egg and sperm (also called fertilization)

Cord-blood stem cells: cells found in umbilical-cord blood and which have the potential to form different types of cell

Cybrid (human-animal): an embryo created by Somatic Cell Nuclear Transfer (also called Cytoplasmic (human-animal) hybrid embryo)

Cytoplasm: the gel-like substance enclosed in the main body of the cell outside the cell nucleus

DNA (deoxyri-bonucleic acid) sequences: The combination of DNA molecules that make up specific genes

DI: donor insemination

Ectopic pregnancy: a pregnancy within the fallopian tube

Ecology: the study of the relationship between living organisms and their environment

Embryo (human): the organism from the time of fertilization until the end of the eighth week

Embryonic stem cells: early stage embryonic cells with the potential to form a wide range of cell types

Eugenics: the promotion or selection of offspring with specific characteristics

Euthanasia: the intentional killing of a person by an act or omission in order to alleviate suffering

Fallopian tube: the tube between the ovary and the uterus

Fertilization: the union of egg and sperm

Foetus: the developing human being from the eighth week until birth

Gaia: the thin shell of matter (living and dead) surrounding the incandescent interior of the earth, including the earth's surface and atmosphere

Gamete: egg or sperm

Gene therapy: treatment involving transfer of genetic material to cells

Genes: DNA sequences coding for specific proteins and carrying hereditary information

Genetic conditions: hereditary conditions

Genetic enhancement: the promotion of a specific characteristic such as musicality by means of gene technology

Genetically modified organisms (GM organisms): animals or plants that have been genetically altered to promote specific characteristics

Germ-line cells: sperm or egg or cells which will develop into sperm or eggs (including the cells of the early embryo)

Germ-line gene therapy: transfer of genetic material to germ-line cells

Human-animal chimeras: human embryos containing animal cells added to them during early development

Human genome: the complete set of genetic material of an individual human

Human-animal (or animal-human) hybrid: an organism with both human and animal genes (DNA) in every cell.

Hybrid: an organism with genes from two or more species within all their cells

Implantation: the attachment of the embryo to the lining of the uterus

IUI: intra-uterine insemination

IVF (*in vitro* fertilization): fertilization in a glass dish

Mitochondria: energy-producing structures in the cytoplasm of cells

Mitochondrial diseases: disorders relating to mitochondrial genes

Mitochondrial genes: genes (DNA) within mitochondria

Monozygotic twinning: the division of one embryo into two embryos

Mutation: a spontaneous genetic change

Nuclear genome: the genes (DNA) carried on the chromosomes within the cell nucleus

Nucleus: the part of the cell containing the chromosomes

Physician-assisted suicide: the provision by a doctor of the means whereby the patient can kill himself

Placenta: the foetal organ from which the foetus receives its nourishment from the mother

Pluripotent: the ability of cells (e.g. embryonic stem cells) to develop into different types of cell and tissue

Predictive testing: testing of a person to diagnose a late-onset genetic condition that may affect the individual in the future

Pre-implantation diagnosis: testing of the IVF embryo to diagnose a genetic condition

Pre-implantation screening: testing of the IVF embryo to diagnose a chromosomal condition (such as Down syndrome)

Prenatal screening: testing to see whether the foetus is at risk of being affected by a medical condition

Prenatal diagnosis: diagnosis of medical condition in the foetus

Primitive streak: a structure in the embryo developing around 14 days after fertilization

Renewable energy: energy generated by the sun, the wind or other sources that may be tapped indefinitely

Saviour sibling: an IVF embryo created to serve as a tissue donor for a sick sibling

Somatic Cell Nuclear Transfer (SCNT): the transfer of the nucleus of an adult somatic cell (such as a skin cell) into an egg from which the nucleus has been removed (also called cloning)

Somatic gene therapy: transfer of genetic material to body cells in order to cure an individual of a disease

Stem cells: cells which can continuously divide to produce identical cells and which also have the ability to produce specialized cells (such as blood or skin cells)

Therapeutic cloning: the creation of embryos by SCNT to produce embryonic stem cells genetically matched to a particular person. (The aim is to find treatment for a variety of diseases.)

Transgenic organism: a hybrid created by transplanting DNA (genes) from one species to another

True human-animal hybrid embryo: an embryo created by fertilizing a human egg with animal sperm or an animal egg with human sperm

Umbilical cord: the cord transporting blood from the placenta to the foetus

Xenotransplantation: organ or tissue transplantation from one species to another

Zygote: the one-cell embryo

NOTES

2. THE BEGINNING OF LIFE

1 While the 1990 Act will be amended to keep up with scientific developments, the 14-day limit for human embryo research is set to remain.
What is changing is the definition of an embryo, which is being widened
to include not only the fertilized egg, but also 'an egg that is in the
process of fertilization or is undergoing any other process capable of
resulting in an embryo' (Human Fertilization and Embryology Bill
2007).

2 Cf., Brent Waters, who writes: 'A significant threshold is reached at
implantation, for with gestation there is a relationship between child and
parents that did not exist previously. During pregnancy there is mutual
disclosing of this relationship, and a covenant of familial fidelity is initiated' (Waters, 2001: 123).

3 David Albert Jones has provided a detailed account of the Christian tradition and its views on animation. See, Jones, 2004.

4 See Fletcher, 1974: 147–87.

5 See *Report of the Committee of Inquiry into Human Fertilization and
Embryology* (Warnock Report, 1984).

6 In this group were Dr Anne McLaren, the embryologist on the Warnock
Committee and Dr Penelope Leach a member of the Voluntary
Licensing Committee preceding the HFEA, set up under the HFE Act
1990. The Ethics Committee of the American Fertility Society also
advanced this type of argument. The Australian Jesuit theologian
Norman Ford did so too, but he did not endorse embryo research.

7 Anne McLaren, the embryologist on the Warnock Committee, used the
word 'toti-potent' (McLaren, 1986). Penelope Leach, a member of the
Voluntary Licensing Authority, preceding the HFEA, used the term
'undifferentiated' (Leach, 1985). The Ethics Committee of the American
Fertility Society (AFS) favoured the term 'full developmental potential'
(American Fertility Society, 1986).

8 Cf., Singer *et al.*, 1990.

9 With the advance of science, it may be possible to observe monozygotic

twinning before the appearance of the primitive streak. But this does not change the fact that the number of primitive streaks observed shows how many embryos there are. Nor does it change the logic of the argument.

10 The Warnock Committee explicitly recognized this at the same time as it emphasized that there is a discontinuity regarding individual identity in the case of twinning.

3. RESPECT FOR HUMAN LIFE AND PERSONHOOD

1 Others who argue on these lines are, for example, Joseph Fletcher (Fletcher, 1954), Jonathan Glover (Glover, 1977), Michael Tooley (Tooley, 1983) and John Harris (Harris, 1985).

4. ABORTION: QUALITY *VERSUS* SANCTITY OF LIFE

1 Nigel M. de S. Cameron is another bioethicist much concerned with contemporary challenges to the Hippocratic ethos and ethics of medicine (Cameron, 2001).
2 Up-to-date statistics can be found at www.dh.gov.uk.

5. EUTHANASIA: QUALITY *VERSUS* SANCTITY OF LIFE

1 Arguably, the UK's Mental Capacity Act 2005, discussed below, represents another step in the direction of legalizing euthanasia by omission.
2 Wyatt's definition of letting die is very similar to that of John Paul II (John Paul II, 1995, para. 65).
3 This point is well made by Stanley Hauerwas in his work, *Suffering Presence* (Hauerwas, 1986).

6. REPRODUCTIVE TECHNOLOGIES AND CLONING

1 Data relating to fertility treatment can be obtained on the HFEA website.
2 For other Christian interventions in the debate see, notably, Brendan McCarthy's collection (McCarthy, 1997).
3 Donor anonymity has also been abolished in Sweden, Norway, The Netherlands, New Zealand and parts of Australia.
4 In Alexandra McWhinnie's book, three donor conceived adults tell us about their searches for their genetic parents and intense longings to know their genetic roots (McWhinnie, 2006).
5 The same would apply if the treatment involved sperm donation.
6 The first IVF baby from a frozen and thawed embryo was born to a couple in Australia in 1984 (HFEA, 2005: 2).

7 For a long time this put the UK in a unique position in Europe. This was not least because the 1997 Bioethics Convention of the Council of Europe – which sanctioned embryo research in countries whose national legislation allowed it – banned the creation of embryos expressly for research purposes. Even today most European countries only allow embryo research using embryos left over after IVF.

8 K. Takahshi *et al.*, 2007, 'Induction of Pluripotent Stem Cells from Adult Human Fibroblasts by Defined Factors', *Cell* 131: 1–12.; J. Yu *et al.*, 2007, 'Induced Pluripotent Stem Cell Lines Derived from Human Somatic Cells' www.sciencemag.org/cgi/content/abstract/1151526.

9 In February 2005, the United Nations rejected both reproductive and therapeutic cloning, mainly on the ground that cloning requires a vast amount of eggs and could lead to the exploitation of women.

10 The technique in question has been pioneered in the UK at the Centre for Sight, at Queen Victoria Hospital in East Grinstead. Information can be found on the hospital's website.

11 The legal status of this procedure seems presently unclear in the UK, but the procedure is set to become explicitly legalized. See Human Fertilization and Embryology Bill 2007.

12 The BSR had also presented an earlier submission to the Warnock Committee in March 1983 making the same substantial points as in the 1984 report.

13 For example, Brent Waters distinguishes between the attitude of 'procreative stewardship' which is protective of nascent human life and the attitude of 'procreative liberty' which has coloured an ever increasingly instrumental attitude towards the unborn child (Waters, 2001).

7. GENETICS, EUGENICS AND INSTRUMENTALISM

1 Twenty-five years after Lewis voiced his warning, but equally concerned about genetic engineering of the future, Paul Ramsey expressed the fear that we would take control over the next stage of human evolution (Ramsey, 1970a: 152).

2 Useful information on PGD and screening in connection with IVF can be obtained on the HFEA website.

3 The ethos spoken of comes to the fore not least in the cost-benefit analysis studies of genetic services that are regularly published in medical journals and elsewhere, as is reluctantly recognized by the UK's Human Genetics Commission (HGC), when it admits that 'cost-benefit analyses of genetic services can be contentious if they entail a crude monetary valuation being placed on the lives of individuals with particular genetic conditions' (HGC, 2006, para, 6.12). The document is available on www.hgc.gov.uk.

4 Recognizing these kinds of concern, the HGC has recommended not only systematic medical follow-up for all such children but also research into their wellbeing (HGC, 2006, para. 4.22).

5 Useful information may be found on www.hgc.gov.uk and on http://genome.wellcome.ac.uk.
6 See Report of the Committee on the Ethics of Gene Therapy (the Clothier Report) 1992.

8. ORGAN TRANSPLANTATION, HYBRIDS AND CHIMERAS

1 See, David Hill, 'Is Brainstem Death Diagnostic or Merely Prognostic? And Does it Matter? , *Triple Helix*, Spring 1999: 4–6.
2 Expressing grave doubts, David Albert Jones says that the patient's body may still be alive when a patient is declared brain dead (Jones, 2001: 52–61). And Leon Kass says, 'the primary stimulus to seek a new definition of death was the need for organs for transplantation' (Kass, 1985: 30).
3 The regulator in these countries is the Human Tissue Authority (HTA), established in 2004.
4 Thus, as explained in the Human Tissue Authority's Code of Practice, reimbursement for expenses and lost earnings only is allowed. And this is provided that the expenses are paid by a proper authority such as an NHS Trust or a foundation hospital and not by the recipients or his or her family or friends (HTA, 2006, paras. 63–5).
5 The BioCentre has produced a detailed report on hybrids and chimeras. The report, which was prepared by a working party chaired by Calum MacKellar, Director of Research at the Scottish Council on Human Bioethics, was addressed to the House of Lords and House of Commons Joint Committee on the Draft Human Tissue and Embryo Bill, published 17 May 2007 (MacKellar, 2007). The report can be downloaded from: www.bioethics.ac.uk.
6 See Human Fertilization and Embryology Bill 2007.
7 See MacKellar, 2007.

10. HOW TO TREAT AND NOT TO TREAT ANIMALS

1 James Watson is the Nobel laureate who discovered the structure of DNA.
2 Another proponent of animal rights is Tom Regan, who argues that it takes no more than reason to recognize that animals have rights, 'because they have intrinsic value', because they are 'experiencing subjects of life' (Regan, 1989: 108).
3 Scott Bader-Saye, speaks of Augustine's and Aquinas' instrumental attitudes towards animals (Bader-Saye, 2001: 3); James Gaffney too speaks regretfully about the Christian tradition (Gaffney, 1998: 100–2).
4 Information about UK regulations concerning animal welfare can be found on DEFRA's website.
5 See www.grain.org/go/birdflu.
6 See www.rds-online.org.uk.

7 Statistics and information relating to animal research may be obtained on the Home Office website at: www.homeoffice.gov.uk/science-research/animal-testing.

11. ECOLOGY AND THE GUARDIANS OF CREATION

1 Cf., Celia Deane-Drummond, *Creation through Wisdom: Theology and the New Biology* (London: T&T Clark, 2000). This work explores the biblical wisdom literature in order to apply it to our thinking on attitudes to the living world.

BIBLIOGRAPHY

American Fertility Society (1986): 'Ethical Consideration on the New Reproductive Technology', *Fertility and Sterility* 46, Suppl. 1.

Aquinas (1964–1976): St Thomas Aquinas: *Summa Theologiae* (ST) (trans. T. Gilby and T. C. O'Brien (eds); 60 vols; London and New York: Blackfriars, in conjunction with Eyre & Spottiswood and McGraw-Hill Book Company).

— (1956) *Summa Contra Gentiles* (ScG) (trans. A. C. Pegis *et al.*; Garden City, NJ: Doubleday, 2nd edn.).

Aristotle (1946): *Politics of Aristotle* (trans. with an introduction, notes and appendices by E. Barker; Oxford: Oxford University Press).

Ashley B. M., and K. D. O'Rourke (1989): *Healthcare Ethics: A Theological Analysis* (St Louis, MO: The Catholic Health Association of the United States).

Bacon, F. (1989): *New Atlantis* (J. Weinberger (ed.); Wheeling, IL: Harlan Davidson, revised edn.).

Bader-Saye, S. (2000) 'Imaging God through Peace with Animals', *Studies in Christian Ethics* 14, no. 2: 1–13.

Baliey, L. L., S. L. Nehlsen-Cannarella, W. Conception, and W. B. Jolley (1985): 'Baboon to Human Cardiac Xenographic Transplantation in a Neonate', *Journal of the American Medical Association* 254: 3321–9.

Banner, M. (1999): *Christian Ethics and Contemporary Moral Problems* (Cambridge: Cambridge University Press).

Barth, K. (1961): *Church Dogmatics*, III. 4, G. W. Bromiley and T. F. Torrance (eds) (Edinburgh: T & T Clark).

Basil the Great (1984) *Basil the Great: Letter to Amphilochus concerning the Canons*, Ep. 188, in P. Schaff and H. Wace (eds), *Nicene and Post-Nicene Fathers*, vol. 8 (trans. with notes by B. Jackson; Edinburgh and Grand Rapids, MI: T&T Clark and Eerdmans, 2nd series): 223–8.

Beauchamp T. L., and J. F. Childress (2001): *Principles of Biomedical Ethics: Fifth Edition* (Oxford: Oxford University Press).

Berry, R. (2000): *The Care of Creation* (Leicester: IVP).

Board for Social Responsibility (BSR) (1984): *Human Fertilization and Embryology: The Response of the Board for Social Responsibility of the*

General Synod of the Church of England to the DHSS Report of the Committee of Inquiry (London: BSR).

Board of Social Responsibility, *Personal Origins* (1985): *The Report of a Working Party on Human Fertilization and Embryology of the Board of Social Responsibility* (London: CIO Publishing).

Boethius (1891): *Liber de Persona et Duabus Naturis: Contra Eutychen et Nestorium* (LP), in J.-P. Migne (ed.), *Patrologia Latina*, vol. 64 (Paris: Apud Garnier Frates Editions et J.-P. Migne Successores).

Broberg, G., and N. Roll-Hansen (1996): *Eugenics and the Welfare State Sterilization Policy in Denmark, Sweden, Norway and Finland* (East Lansing: Michigan State University Press).

Brody, B. (1975): *Abortion and the Sanctity of Human Life: A Philosophical View* (Cambridge, MA: MIT Press).

Bryant, J., and P. Turnpenny (2003): 'Genetics and Genetic Modification of Humans: Principles, Practice and Possibilities', in C. Deane-Drummond (ed.), *Brave New World? Theology, Ethics and the Human Genome* (London: T&T Clark): 5–26.

Cameron, N. M. de S. (2001): *The New Medicine: Life and Death after Hippocrates* (Chicago and London: Bioethics Press).

Campbell, A., G. Gillett, and G. Jones. (2001): *Medical Ethics* (Oxford: Oxford University Press, 3rd edn.).

Catechism of the Catholic Church (1999): (New York: Burns & Oates).

Catholic Bishops' Conference of England and Wales (2002): *The Call of Creation* (London: Catholic Bishops' Conference of England and Wales).

Catholic Bishops' Joint Committee on Bioethical Issues on Behalf of the Catholic Bishops of Great Britain (1983): *In Vitro Fertilisation and Public Policy: Evidence Submitted to the Government Committee of Inquiry into Human Fertilization and Embryology* (London: Catholic Media Office).

Catholic Bishop's Joint Committee on Bio-Ethical Issues (1984): *Response to the Warnock Report on Human Fertilization and Embryology* (London: Catholic Media Office).

Charlesworth, M. (1989): *Life, Death, Genes and Ethics* (Crows Nest, NSW: ABC Book).

Clothier, C. (Chair) (1992): *The Report of the Committee on the Ethics of Gene Therapy* (London: HMSO).

Congregation for the Doctrine of the Faith (CDF) (1986): *Respect for Human Life in Its Origin and the Dignity of Procreation (Donum Vitae)* (Vatican City: Libreria Editrice Vaticana).

Congregation for the Doctrine of the Faith (2007): *Responses to Certain Questions of the USCCB (United States Conference of Catholic Bishops) concerning Artificial Nutrition and Hydration* (Vatican City: Libreria Editrice Vaticana).

Cooper, D. K., A. Dorling, P. N. Pierson, N. Richard, M. Rees, M. J. Seebach, M. Yazer, H. Ohdan, M. Awwad and D. Ayares (2007): *Transplantation* 84, Issue 1: 1–7.

Council of Europe (1997): *Convention for the Protection of Human Rights and Dignity of the Human Being with regard to the Application of Biology and Medicine: Convention on Human Rights and Biomedicine* (Ovideo: Council of Europe).

— (2005): *Additional Protocol to the Convention on Human Rights and Bioemedicine concerning Biomedical Research* (Strasbourg: Council of Europe).

Curran, C. (1975): *Ongoing Revision: Studies in Moral Theology* (Notre Dame: University of Notre Dame Press).

Dainiak, N., and R. C. Ricks (2005): 'The Evolving Role of Haematopoietic Cell Transplantation in Radiation Injury: Potentials and Limitations', *The British Journal of Radiology Supplement* 27: 169–74.

Daly, T. V. (1987): 'NSW Law Reform Commission Invites Discussion on the Embryo', *St Vincent Bioethics Centre Newsletter* 5, no. 3: 11.

Darwin, C. (1996): *The Origin of the Species* (with an introduction and notes by G. Beer (ed.); Oxford: Oxford University Press).

Deane-Drummond, C. (2002): *Creation through Wisdom: Theology and the New Biology* (London: T&T Clark).

Deane-Drummond, C. (ed.) (2003): *Brave New World? Theology, Ethics and the Human Genome* (London: T&T Clark).

Department of Health (2004a): *Statutory Instrument 2004 No. 1031, The Medicines for Human Use (Clinical Trials) Regulations 2004* (London: Department of Health).

— (2004b) *The Human Tissue Act 2004* (London: Department of Health).

— (2006a) *Xenotransplantation Guidance* (London: Department of Health).

— (2006b) *Human Tissues and Embryos (Draft) Bill* (London: Department of Health).

Descartes, R. (1972): *Meditations of the First Philosophy, in Descartes Philosophical Writings* (trans. E. Anscombe and P. T. Geach (eds); London: Nelson's University Press).

Doherty, P. (ed.) (1995): *Post-Abortion Syndrome: Its Wide Ramifications* (Dublin: Four Courts Press).

Doherty, P., and A. Sutton (eds) (1998): *Man-Made Man: Ethical and Legal Issues in Genetics* (Dublin: Open Air Press).

Dunstan, G. R. (1988): 'The Human Embryo in the Western Moral Tradition', in G. R. Dunstan and M. Sellar (eds), *The Status of the Human Embryo: Perspectives from Moral Tradition* (London: King's Fund): 39–57.

Dworkin, R. (1995): *Life's Dominion* (New York: HarperCollins).

Engelhart, T., Jr. (1986): *The Foundations of Bioethics* (Oxford: Oxford University Press).

European Parliament and Council (2001): Directive 2001/20/EC of the European Parliament and Council, *Official Journal of the European Community*, L121 2001, pp. 34–44.

Fisher, A., and M. Cavazzana-Calvo (2006): 'Whither Gene Therapy', *The Scientist*, 20, Issue 2: 36–43.

Fletcher, J. (1954): *Morals and Medicine* (Boston, MA: The Beacon Press).

— (1974) *The Ethics of Genetic Control* (Garden City, NY: Anchor Books).

Ford, N. M. (1988): *When Did I Begin?* (Cambridge: Cambridge University Press).

Fukuyama, F. (2002): *Our Posthuman Future: Consequences of the Biotechnology Revolution* (London: Profile Books).

Galton, F. (1904): 'Eugenics: Its Definition, Scope and Aims', *The American Journal of Sociology* 10, no. 1: 1–2.

Glover, J. (1977): *Causing Death and Saving Lives* (Harmondsworth: Penguin Books).

Goethe (1959): *Faust*, Part 2 (trans. with an introduction by P. Wayne; Harmondsworth: Penguin Books).

Gunton, C. (1996): *The Promise of Trinitarian Theology* (London: T&T Clark, 2nd edn.).

Häring, B. (1976): 'New Dimension in Responsible Parenthood', *Theological Studies* 37: 122–32.

Harris, J. (1985): *The Value of Life: An Introduction to Medical Ethics* (London, Boston, Melbourne and Henley: Routledge & Kegan Paul).

Hauerwas, S. (1986): *Suffering Presence: Theological Reflections on Medicine, the Mentally Handicapped, and the Church* (Edinburgh: T&T Clark).

HFEA (2005) *Annual Report: Facing the Future, 2004–5* (London: HFEA).

H.M. Treasury (2007): *Stern Review on the Economics of Climate Change* (London: H.M. Treasury).

Hoedemaerkers, R. and Have H. ten (1987): 'Geneticization: The Cyprus Paradigm', *Journal of Medicine and Philosophy* 23: 279–80.

Holy Bible, English Standard Version (2002) (London: Collins).

House of Commons Science and Technology Committee (2004): *Fifth Report of Session 2004–05: Human Reproductive Technologies and the Law* (London: HMSO).

House of Lords (2007): Human Fertilization and Embryology Bill [HL] 2007.

Human Genetics Commission (HGC) (2005): *Making Babies: Reproductive Decisions and Genetic Technologies* (London: Human Genetics Commission).

Human Tissue Authority (HTA) (2006): *Code of Practice – Donation of Organs, Tissue and Cells for Transplantation* (London: Human Tissue Authority).

Huxley, A. (2004): *Brave New World* (with an introduction by D. Bradshaw; London: Vintage).

Iglesias, T. (1988): 'In Vitro Fertilisation: The Major Issues', in N. M. de S. Cameron (ed.), *Embryos and Ethics* (Edinburgh: Rutherford House Books): 14–27.

Intergovernmental Panel on Climate Change (IPCC), Working Group I (2007): *Fourth Assessment Report: Climate Change 2007: The Physical Science Basis* (Geneva: IPCC).

Intergovernmental Panel on Climate Change, Working Group II (2007): *Fourth Assessment Report: Climate Change 2007: Climate Change Impacts, Adaptation and Vulnerability* (Geneva: IPCC).

Intergovernmental Panel on Climate Change, Working Group III (2007) *Fourth Assessment Report: Climate Change 2007: Mitigation of Climate Change* (Geneva: IPCC).

John Paul II (1995): Encyclical Letter, *Evangelium Vitae* (Vatican City: Libreria Vaticana).

— (1997) *The Theology of the Body: Human Love in the Divine Plan* (Boston: Pauline Books and Media).

Jones, D. (2001): *Organ Transplants* (London: Catholic Truth Society and Linacre Centre).

— (2004) *The Soul of the Embryo* (London, New York: Continuum).

Jonsen, A. R. (2003): *The Birth of Bioethics* (Oxford: Oxford University Press).

Kant, I. (1998): *Groundwork of the Metaphysics of Morals*, M. Gregor (ed.) (Cambridge: Cambridge University Press).

Kass L. R. (1985): *Toward a More Natural Science* (New York: The Free Press).

Kelly, G. (1956): 'The Morality of Mutilation: Towards a Revision of the Treatise', *Theological Studies* 17, no. 3: 322–44.

Keown, J. (1992): 'Some Reflections on Euthanasia in the Netherlands', in L. Gormally (ed.), *The Dependent Elderly: Autonomy, Justice and Quality of Care* (Cambridge: Cambridge University Press): 70–100.

— (2002) *Euthanasia, Ethics and Public Policy* (Cambridge: Cambridge University Press).

Kilner J. F., N. M. de S. Cameron, and S, Schniedermayer (eds) (1995): *Bioethics and the Future: A Christian Appraisal* (Grand Rapids, MI: W. B. Eerdmans Publishing Co.).

King, D. (1996): 'Eugenic Tendencies in Modern Genetics', in P. Doherty and A. Sutton (eds), *Man-Made Man: Ethical and Legal Issues in Genetics* (Dublin: Open Air Press): 71–82.

King, U. (2006): 'One Planet, One Spirit: Searching for an Ecologically Balanced Spirituality', in *Ecotheology: The Journal of Religion, Nature and the Environment* 10, no. 1: 66–87.

Kuehnle, I., and M. A. Goodell (2002): 'The Therapeutic Potential of Stem Cells from Adults', *British Medical Journal* 325: 372–6.

Kuhse, H. (1996): 'Voluntary Euthanasia and Other Medical End-of-Life Decisions: Doctors should be Permitted to give Death a Helping Hand', in D. C. Thomasma and T. Kushner (eds), *Birth to Death: Science and Bioethics* (Cambridge: Cambridge University Press): 247–58.

Kuhse, H., and P. Singer (1985): *Should the Baby Live? The Problem of Handicapped Infants* (Oxford: Oxford University Press).

Junying, Y. *et al.* (2006): 'Induced Pluripotent Stem Cell Lines derived from Human Somatic Cells', *Science*, www.sciencemag.org/cgi/content/abstract/1151526

Leach, P. (1985): *First Report of the Licensing Authority for Human Fertilization and Embryology*, Annex 3 (London: HMSO).

Lennard. A. L., and G. H. Jackson (2000): 'Science, Medicine and the Future: Stem cell Transplantation', *British Medical Journal* 321: 433–7.

Lewis, C. S. (1989): 'Vivisection', in S. Lammers and A. Verhey (eds), *On Moral Medicine: Theological Perspectives in Medical Ethics* (Grand Rapids, MI: Eerdmans): 597–8.

— (2001): *The Abolition of Man* (New York: HarperSanFrancisco).

Lifton, R. J. (1986): *The Nazi Doctors: A Study in the Psychology of Evil* (London: Papermac, 3rd edn.).

Linzey, A. (1976): 'The Theos-Rights of Animals', in T. Regan and P. Singer (eds), *Animal Rights and Human Obligations* (Englewoods Cliffs, NJ: Prentice-Hall, 2nd edn.): 134–48.

— (1987) *Christianity and the Rights of Animals* (London: SPCK).

— (2002a) 'Animal Rights: A Reply to Barclay', in N. Messer (ed.), *Theological Issues in Bioethics: An Introduction with Readings* (London: Darton, Longman and Todd): 223–7.

— (2002b) 'An Open Letter to the Bishops on Hunting', *Church Times* (20 Dec.).

Linzey, A. and D. Cohn-Sherbok (1997): *After Noah: Animals and the Liberation of Theology* (London: Mowbray).

Linzey, A. and D. Yamamoto (1988): *Animals on the Agenda* (London: SCM Press).

Locke, J. (2004): *Essay Concerning Human Understanding*, R. Woolhouse (ed.) (London: Penguin Classics).

Lovelock, J. (2006): *The Revenge of Gaia* (London: Allen Lane).

Lucas, C. (2006): *Avian Flu: Time to Shut the Intensive Poultry 'Flu Factories'?* (Brussels: The Greens and EFA, European Parliament).

MacKellar, C. (Chair) (2007): *BioCentre Report: The New Inter-Species Future? An Ethical Discussion of Embryonic, Fetal and Post-natal Human-Nonhuman Combinations* (London: BioCentre).

McCarthy, B. (1998): *Fertility & Faith: The Ethics of Human Fertilization* (Leicester: Inter Varsity Press).

McCormick, R. (1981): *How Brave a New World? Dilemmas in Bioethics* (London: SCM Press).

McGrath, A. E. (2002): 'The Stewardship of Creation: An Evangelical Affirmation', in R. J. Berry (ed.) *The Care of Creation* (Leicester: InterVarsity Press): 86–9.

McLaren, A. (1986): 'Prelude or Embryogenesis', in G. Brock and M. O'Connor (eds), *Human Embryo Research, Yes or No?* (London: Ciba Foundation).

McLean, J. (1977): 'Embryogenesis of Monozygotic Twins', *Catholic Medical Quarterly* 41, no. 2: 65–72.

McWhinnie, A. (2006): *Who am I?* (Leamington Spa: Idreos Education Trust).

Malthus, T. (1798): *An Essay on the Principle of Population, as it Affects the Future Improvement of Society* (London).

Meilaender, G. (1996): *Bioethics: A Primer for Christians* (Grand Rapids, MI: Eerdmans).

Messer, N. (ed.) (2002): *Theological Issues in Bioethics: An Introduction with Readings* (London: DLT).

Miles, S. H. (2004): *The Hippocratic Oath and the Ethics of Medicine* (Oxford: Oxford University Press).

Naess, A. (1990): *Ecology, Community and Lifestyle* (Cambridge: Cambridge University Press).

Nuremberg Code (1947): Reprinted from *Trials of War Criminals before the Nuremberg Military Tribunals under Control Council Law* (Washington, DC: US Government Printing Office), no. 10, vol. 2, pp. 181–2.

Nys H. (2007): 'European Biolaw in the Making', in C. Gastmans, K. Dierickx, H. Nys and P. Schotsmans (eds), *New Pathways for European Bioethics* (Antwerp and Oxford: Intersentia): 161–78.

O'Donovan, O. (1984): *Begotten or Made?* (Oxford: Clarendon Press).

Paul VI (1968): Encyclical Letter *Humanae Vitae* (London: Catholic Truth Society).

Piotrowska, K., and M. Zernicka-Goetz (2001): 'Role for Sperm in Spatial Patterning of the Early Mouse Embryo', *Nature* 409: 517–21.

Piotrowska, K., F. Wianny, R. A., Pedersen, and M. Zernicka-Goetz (2001): 'Blastomeres Arising from the First Cleavage Division have Distinguishable Fates in Normal Mouse Development', *Development* 128: 3739–48.

Plato (1941): *The Republic of Plato*, trans. with an introduction and notes by F. MacDonald Cornford (Oxford: Oxford University Press).

Rahner, K. (1972): 'The Problem of Genetic Manipulation', in *Theological Investigations*, vol. 9 (London: Darton, Longman & Todd): 244–52.

Ramsey, P. (1968): 'The Morality of Abortion', in D. H. Labby (ed.), *Life or Death: Ethics and Options* (Washington: University of Washington Press).

— (1970) *Fabricated Man* (New Haven and London: Yale University Press).

— (1975) *The Patient as a Person: Explanations in Medical Ethics* (New Haven: Yale University Press).

Regan T. (1976) 'The Case for Animal Rights', in T. Regan and P. Singer (eds), *Animal Rights and Human Obligations* (Englewood Cliffs, NJ: Prentice Hall): 105–14.

Riddle, J. M. (1994) *Contraception and Abortion from the Ancient World to the Renaissance* (Cambridge, MA: Harvard University Press).

Rosenthal N. (2003) 'Prometheus's Vulture and the Stem-Cell Promise', *The New England Journal of Medicine* 349: 267–74.

Saunders, C. (1990): 'Euthanasia: The Hospice Alternative', in N. M. de S. Cameron (ed.), *Death without Dignity* (Edinburgh: Rutherford House Books): 196–205.

Serra, A. (1992): 'The Human Embryo, Science and Medicine: Commentary on a Recent Document', in J.-F. Malherbe (ed.), *Human Life, its Beginnings and Development: Bioethical Reflections by Catholic Scholars* (Louvain-la-Neuve: Ciaco): 39–52.

Silver, L. (2007): *Remaking Eden: How Genetic Engineering and Cloning will Transform the American Family* (London: HarperCollins, 2nd edn.).

Singer, P. (1976): 'All Animals are Equal', in T. Regan and P. Singer (eds), *Animal Rights and Human Obligations* (Englewood Cliffs, NJ: Prentice-Hall): 73–86.

Singer, P. (1995a) *Rethinking Life and Death* (Oxford: Oxford University Press).

— (1995b) *Animal Liberation* (London: Pimlico, 2nd edn.).

Singer, P., H. Kuhse, S. Buckle, K., Dawson, and P. Kasimba (1992): *Embryo Experimentation: Ethical, Legal and Social Issues* (Cambridge: Cambridge University Press).

Song, R. (2002): *Human Genetics: Fabricating the Future* (London: Darton, Longman and Todd).

Sutton, A. (1990): *Prenatal Diagnosis: Confronting the Ethical Issues* (London: The Linacre Centre).

— (1995) 'Abortion: Psychological Indications and Consequences', in P. Doherty (ed.), *Post-Abortion Syndrome: Its Wide Implications* (Dublin: Four Courts Press).

— (2007) 'Saviour Siblings', *Medicina e Morale* 6: 1179–88.

Takahashi, K., *et al.* (2007): 'Induction of Pluripotent Stem Cells from Adult Human Fibroblasts by Defined Factors', *Cell* 131, 1–12.

Teilhard de Chardin, P. (1978): 'The Mass of the World', in P. Teilhard de Chardin, *The Heart of Matter*, trans. R. Hague (London: Collins): 119–34.

Tertullian (1997a): *Apology*, in A. Roberts and J. Donaldson (eds), *Ante-Nicene Fathers*, vol. 3 (Chronologically arranged and with brief notes and preface by A. Cleveland Coxe D.D.; Edinburgh and Grand Rapids, MI: T&T Clark and Eerdmans, American reprint of the Edinburgh edition): 2–55.

Tertullian (1997b): *Against Praxeas*, in A. Roberts and J. Donaldson (eds), *Ante-Nicene Fathers*, vol. 3 (Chronologically arranged with brief notes and preface by A. Cleveland Coxe D.D.: Edinburgh and Grand Rapids, MI: T&T Clark and Eerdmans, American reprint of the Edinburgh edition): 597–628.

Thomasma, D. C., and T. Kushner (eds) (1996): *Birth to Death: Science and Bioethics* (Cambridge: Cambridge University Press).

Tonti-Fillippini, N. (1987): 'Further Comments on the Beginning of Life', *Linacre Quarterly* 59, no. 3: 76–81.

Tooley, M. (1983): *Abortion and Infanticide* (Oxford: Oxford University Press).

UNESCO (2005): *Universal Declaration on Bioethics and Human Rights* (New York: UNESCO).

Warnock, M. (1999): *Making Babies: Is there a Right to have Children?* (Oxford: Oxford University Press).

Warnock, M. (Chair) (1984): *Report of the Committee of Inquiry into Human Fertilization and Embryology* (London: HMSO).

Waters, B. (1998): *Reproductive Technology: Towards a Theology of Procreative Stewardship* (London: Darton, Longman and Todd).

Watt, H. (1999): *Life and Death in Healthcare Ethics: A Short Introduction* (London: Routledge).

Wilmut, I. *et al.* (1997): 'Viable Offspring derived from Foetal and Adult Mammalian Cells', *Nature* 385: 810–13.

World Health Organization (WHO) (2003): EB112, 5 (Geneva: WHO).

World Medical Association (1957): *Principles for Those in Research and Experimentation* (Ferney-Voltaire: WMA).

— (1964) *Declaration of Helsinki* (several times amended and with added notes of clarification; Tokyo: WMA, 2004).

— (1970) *Declaration of Oslo: Statement on Therapeutic Abortion* (Geneva: WMA).

— (2006) *World Medical Association Statement on Human Organ Donation and Transplantation* (Ferney-Voltaire: WMA).
Wyatt, J. (1998): *Matters of Life and Death* (Leicester: Inter Varsity Press).

WEBSITES

www.Defra.gov.uk
www.dh.gov.uk
www.foe.co.uk
www.grain.org
www.hm.treasurey.gov.uk.
www.homeoffice.gov.uk
www.ipcc.ch
www.royalsoc.ac.uk
www. rds-online.org.uk
www.uk-legislation.hmso.gov.uk
www.wwf.org.uk

INDEX